Intentional Wellness

Create Your Optimal Life Now

Intentional Wellness

Create Your Optimal Life Now

by
Sheila Z. Stirling

Wisdom Press

Intentional Wellness: Create Your Optimal Life Now

by Sheila Z. Stirling

Copyright © 2007 Sheila Z. Stirling
ISBN 978-0-9778891-2-9

Published Spring 2008

Published by:

Wisdom Press
4132 S. Rainbow Blvd. #465,
Las Vegas NV, 89103
Phone: (702) 499-4408
Website: www.intentional-wellness.com

Note from the author and publisher: The information in this book is not meant in any way to be or to replace medical advice or treatment.

To order more copies of this book, please contact Wisdom Press at www.wisdompresspublishing.com

www.wisdompresspublishing.com

Edited and designed by Tony Stubbs, www.tjpublish.com

Cover design by Katlyn Breene

Printed in the United States of America

Table of Contents

Acknowledgments

Where do you start when all of the universe has been pushing and pulling, sending information and visions, and putting the pieces together like a giant 3-D globe?

I am so grateful for every moment and so in awe with this journey. I want to acknowledge everything. I mean everything. The wind, the sun, the moon, the water and precious mother earth. I want to wrap myself around this great place and say thank you.

I want to acknowledge the people in my life whose kindness and support have been like a spring rain to a thirsty tree. That would be Stewart who is so awesome and grounding for me. His love feels like a warm blanket on a cold winter's day. I know our laughter can bring a smile to the whole world. Sometimes he looks at me with amazement and then smiles the smile of acceptance and understanding. How that causes my heart to sing is amazing.

To my close circle – Dwight, Nancy – who are always there to listen, to laugh to help in whatever way they can.

To Anne, who has gone far above and beyond to assist me even if it means burning the midnight oil. I wonder if she knows what an angel she is?

And to the other members of the team – Megan, Juanita and Lea – and all who have helped just by being in my life.

My wonderful daughter, Shane, who is wise beyond her years and to my beautiful grandchildren,– Sage, Elijah and Sierra Pearl – who give me wings to fly.

My sister, Joy, who always has my best interest at heart.

My dear friend Katlyn who is always willing to share her vision and express it with the cover art.

Tony Stubbs, who edits the writing and corrects any misspelled words and believe me, even with spell check, it is a job to correct the spelling.

And then my heart turns to spirit and says thank you for the inspiration, the insight and for sending me the angels. Thank you for the ability to walk in the prayer, to see from a universal perspective and for allowing me to know with certainty that there really is a world of actuality.

For all the readers, seekers, teachers and students, I am so grateful and I acknowledge, validate and love your bright light. Keep it shining always.

About the Author

Although I have known Sheila Z for about one year, sometimes it seems like 10 times that. She has a way of entering into my "space" and seeing things even I didn't know were there. She will drop a comment that reaches deep down where the wound is still raw, crying for healing. Without even knowing or asking, the gift is delivered.

When you watch her interact, as I have on many occasions, with people, it is amazing to witness their reactions. Recently, when Sheila and I were engaged in a conversation, we were approached by a woman who had never met Sheila but had heard of her work. She interrupted our conversation with tears in her eyes and almost pleaded for a moment of Sheila's time. Of course, the intensity was not necessary as Sheila is so gracious about making herself available for those in need of her gifts. My point here is that when the calling is genuine, spirit leads those in need to where the answers are. Sheila is a blessing and a gift to those who know her, both on a professional and a personal level. A gift that becomes more valuable each time there is an opening.

If you have an opportunity to attend one of her workshops or conferences, I encourage you to make every effort you can to be there. In fact, take a friend or two with you. It will be the best gift you could possibly give – to yourself as well as your friends.

Anne Marie
Las Vegas, NV

Preface

The Gift, the Sleep and the Re-awakening

Yes there is a story, there is always a story. Each one of us has a story, a pathway a mountain, whatever our life has shown us or guided us or not guided us. Everyone has a story and this is a very brief synopsis of mine.

Sometimes people ask how and when did I become a healer. For me, the answer goes back to childhood and perhaps beyond that. The gifts revealed to me at such a young age were not understood by me or seen as gifts, but rather felt as sorrow, separation and confusion by such a young spirit.

My story starts when I was very young. I would bring home lost or hurt animals and care for them until they were well. Once when I was about seven, I had a vision that a cat with new kittens was in terrible danger from a dog. I could see it very clearly; I could see the bushes, the hissing cat and the dog drooling, ready to pounce. I could feel the prickly thorns and smell the dust. I ran from the house down the street to the large, empty corner lot. I knew exactly where to run and there, in a corner all covered up with shrubs, was a very scared and hissing cat with her kittens. A large dog was barking and snarling, readying to attack. Without thinking, I grabbed a stick and convinced the dog to go away. I picked up the cat and her kittens and carried them home. I cared for them until they were able to care for themselves. I never stopped to think how I knew where to find the cat and kittens who were in danger. I just knew. I know now I was a visionary at a very young age; perhaps I came in that way (perhaps we all come in that way), seeing events in my mind before they happened or as they were happening.

I drove my mother crazy saving animals of all kinds, and bringing them home. Once I even saved a snail ... a snail! It seems silly now but I remember how serious it was back then, as every creature was so precious to me because I knew somehow that we are all connected. Sometimes if I thought my mom would say no, I would just hide them under my bed and keep it a secret until I could set them free.

Junior High was a wild nightmare for me. I was about 12 and had a vision in which a classmate was hit by a car. I was at home in my bedroom when the vivid image came into me and I felt a wave of pain sweep over my body. Immediately I picked up the phone and called a good friend who lived in the same apartment building as the boy in the vision. I said frantically, "Quick, go tell Pat to stay in for a while. Tell him not to walk to the store."

To my horror, my friend sobbed, "Pat just got hit by a car and the ambulance is taking him away."

Somehow I felt responsible. If I only would have known sooner, maybe I could have stopped it. These visions began to happen more and more, and I isolated myself, feeling that somehow I was different. But then, who at the age of 12 or 13 doesn't feel that way? I wondered, is this the way everyone is? At that time, I felt very alone, afraid to tell anyone about the things I saw.

My parents sent me to summer camp for a few summers and I enjoyed the horses and the activities although I kept to myself most of the time. At the age of 14, I was helping out as a junior camp counselor at a summer camp in California, and had my first encounter with angels. On that bright and sunny summer day, I was on the long, winding path from the dining area (the camp was laid out with the pool, dining room and large recreation area at the top of a hill) down to the cabins. About half way down, I came to the dip in the path when a gust of wind like a dust devil surrounded me. The swirling dust made it hard for me to breathe and I gasped for a breath. Suddenly I felt an angelic presence around me. It felt as if I was being lifted up and held, suspended in time and space. Great wings surrounded me and I was overwhelmed with the love and kindness of those angels that touched my heart and soul. I remember wondering in that moment whether this was what I now know as rapture. I knew *everything and nothing at the same time*. It was as if I was above the world looking down. The whole universe made perfect sense and I felt as if I could heal the wounds of the world, answer any math question or any question at all for that matter. I was in the full stream of consciousness and wanted to stay in that place forever. It felt timeless to me, although it was only a moment in earth time. I didn't realize it then but nothing would ever be the same again for me.

As time went on, the visions became very difficult to manage. For example, one evening I was out with friends in Hollywood and I saw my father having a heart attack. I could feel the pain and see and feel the grimace of disbelief and terror on his face. I raced home and arrived just in time to see the paramedics carrying my father out on a stretcher. I rode in the ambulance with him, with my mother and sister following in the car. No one even asked how I came to be home at just that moment. From that point on, I did whatever it took to cover up the emotional pain and isolation that these visions seemed to bring to me.

Yes, I was a crazy flower child of the 1960s, believing that love and peace would save the world. Come to think of it, I *still* believe that very same thing. By the time I was 18, I felt a deep connection to nature and the great mysteries of this life. and spent as much time as possible in nature. Late in 1968, I went skiing with a friend to Lake Tahoe and didn't return from that trip. I called my mom and said, "Mom, God lives here and I am not leaving."

She said, "Sweetheart, you can't run away from yourself."

I replied, "I know that, mom. I'm not running away, I'm running to."

My parents sent my clothing and the funds I'd saved, and that was that. I never went back to L.A. I was at peace in the high mountains and had a real surge of creativity.

I built my first home at the age of 18 and decided to go into real estate. By 1972, I had a real estate license, a husband and had moved down the mountain to the foothills of the Sierras. I stayed in the corporate world and seemed to be successful at everything I felt compelled to do. When I say 'compelled,' that refers to the ongoing visions and spiritual connection; although it had been pushed to the back burner, it was still always with me. I was an advertising executive and so enjoyed connecting and helping people grow their business.

Through the years, I had many signs to be who I truly was and am. I had moments of deep spiritual connection and clear messages that, "It is time for you to step into your true calling." People were always telling me how they felt peaceful around my energy and sometimes someone would call me an angel. I would smile and think about the angels who came for me so many years earlier. However, I continued to push the gifts away, relating them with my childhood pain and isolation. I was young and stubborn, and not in a listening mood.

Late in 1999, I was given an opportunity to listen 'very closely,' courtesy of an auto accident. It was a beautiful clear night and I was on my way to meet some friends at the Bellagio Hotel in Las Vegas. It was just 10:30 as I looked down at the clock in my brand new custom-made Ford Explorer, four-wheel drive, of course, with sun roof and painted a beautiful, sage green with tan leather interior. (I had been driving Ford Broncos since about 1978 and finally was able to buy my custom 4-door Explorer.) It had only about 3,000 miles on it and I was being careful about my speed so as to be gentle with the engine. I was approaching the intersection of Flamingo and Decatur and looked over to my right, thinking how beautiful the van was just to the right and a little ahead from me. Suddenly, BAM! I never saw what hit me as the van was hit and both vehicles barreled into me. I learned later it was an overworked Pizza Hut driver who'd fallen asleep at the wheel and went into the intersection at full speed.

I was 'taken' once again and given a stern talking to. I was given a choice between staying on the planet and being who I truly am and always had been, live in the prayer that always surrounded me, and be the healer and transmitter I was put here to be ... or I could leave the planet and come back at a later time. Having a grown daughter and two beautiful grandchildren, I chose to stay and wake up. (Little did I know what an effort it would be to fulfill that promise to listen every moment for the rest of my time here.)

I don't really know how long I was out for or gone, but when I came to, the paramedics were on the scene. I awoke holding my head in my hands and begging for forgiveness. I said out loud, "I am so sorry for not listening. I am so sorry. Please don't scream at me anymore."

As the paramedics were about 10 feet away, looking at my car, I received my first instruction … and my first test, although I didn't realize it at the time. "If you go to the hospital with these people, you will not live through the night," were the words I heard in my head and felt in my body.

I did not get out of the car the same person I was when I'd gotten in. I opened my door feeling hot pools running down my face and such a loud buzzing in my head that I couldn't hear. I was numb all over and cold inside. The paramedics said, "You must come with us."

I said, "No, I can't. I'm fine."

They looked at each other and then back at me. Together they said, "NO! You are not fine and you have to come with us."

I just stood there and said, "No! And you cannot force me to go with you."

They said that was true and if I signed some release forms, they would be okay to leave me. So I signed the forms and got a ride from the tow truck driver. (I was not given a clear reason why I could not go to the hospital but I felt it had something to do with the fact that I have allergies to some medications and somehow felt that there would be a fatal error made that night and my opportunity to stay would be very short lived.)

The next few weeks were a blur. I know I went to the doctor the next day for head trauma injuries and had MRIs but to this day, I cannot tell you how I got there or where exactly I went. The bottom line is that among my many physical injuries, I sustained some hefty head and neck injuries, and it really took about three years for me to get to the point where I could converse with people. I experienced isolation like I had never known, and I was thrown into different dimensions, some of them not meant for human viewing. I learned why many people with head trauma choose not to stay. I must confess I understand this feeling very well.

As I was healing, there came a point when I told someone, "In the moment of no more moments, the angels came." (There were times when the severe migraines and the scattered files in my mind were almost too much to bear. There were times I felt if I closed my eyes I would not wake up in this world. It is then that the angels came.) Once again I was shown a clear path on which I was to walk from that point on, and to this day I am so grateful to be at this banquet we call life. I am grateful each and every glorious day. This was my 40 days in the desert, even though it was over 750 days.

As soon as I was able to walk in the world again, I became like a sponge, going to every prophet's conference and seminar, learning many healing modalities. As the saying goes, we teach what we need to learn, and my appetite for knowledge was astounding even to me.

In 2003, I was leaving a seminar when sounds and tones began to come into my mind and my heart. In the weeks that followed, I was visited by angels who gave more of the music and tones to me. I thought *Oh, this is great! I'll use this in my healing practice.*

The tones became louder and louder, until one day I knew I had to get this 'downloaded,' and soon. I called Gary Stadler, a friend in San Diego who has a sound studio and asked him for help. Gary kindly said, "Well, just come on down and let's see what we can do." Thanks to his patience and understanding, note-by-note, the *Sounds of the Soul* came into this dimension, giving a connection with the angels meant to be shared by all.

I have learned that when spirit speaks, *it is to each and every soul*. So here I am, years later and standing in my true shoes. Thanking you for being a part of *Intentional Wellness*. It is the how and why of our optimal self.

Within these pages lie the many facets of wellness, the alchemical mixture that can transform your lead into purest gold. Beyond any secrets and deeper than any rabbit hole. Take in and open your senses, feed the wisdom that awaits your allowing. To feel, see and know your truth, to discover and live your dream is now within your reach. More than that, it is the return to our true liberated and fulfilled self.

This writing is based on and follows the all day Intentional Wellness Conference™ created and offered by Sheila Z Stirling.

Sheila Z

Introduction

Create Your Optimal Life Now
"Live Your Dream"

It is time to share with you my most inner thoughts. When I first started writing *Intentional Wellness*, I pulled another title from a book I started long ago with the intention of using it as a subtitle for *Intentional Wellness*. It is called, *Living the Fountain of Youth*. It is a good, catchy title and just about fits what we are exploring in *Intentional Wellness*. Someday, in the not to distant future, it will come into the world of actuality on its own, but today is not that day. The subtitle must fit like a glove, be right on target and be in total alignment with what Intentional Wellness is sharing and revealing. *Intentional Wellness* is about creating the life you have dreamed. A life of wholeness, wellness and inspiration.

It is now about 3 weeks to the deadline of this book going to print and, as I sit looking out of a very large picture window that sits about 50 feet off the ocean in a small suburb of Vancouver, B.C., it dawned on me that what we are seeking and are now able to grasp is actually the view of life from the universe. So I realized that what this writing may actually be offering you is an opportunity to unravel the mysteries of the perception of the universe. I know this sounds a bit lengthy, with maybe not quite the pizzazz of *Living the Fountain of Youth*, but it is a truer statement and between you and I, there must be only truth.

So what does that really mean? It means there is an inherent order to the universe, that there is the day and the night, the sun and the moon, a season for every stage of life, and death and rebirth. The universe is in continual motion, with every particle and wave of energy constantly moving in a seemingly chaotic state. But the actuality and truth of it is that the universe is not in chaos but in perfect order and harmony. A great symphony is being played out every moment of every moment. The only presence that seems to be in chaos here is us – you and I. In all of this free will over the millennium, just maybe we have overlooked the fact that the universe has put everything here for us. And I *do* mean *everything*. Not only a clue to how the seasons work but also pieces of the puzzle of how to optimize our time here.

We all have everything within us to be fully functioning, in perfect health and perfect wellness – and that means in every aspect of or lives. It is what we came here for. Realizing that we are the divine creation and that the miracle of life lives on in every single one of us is only the beginning of the journey. With physics and spirituality bridging the gap of mere existence, this is the most exciting information in the universe. And the irony is that you already have this information and are fully able to use it to be healthy, wealthy and wise. Therein lies the key word – wisdom, or turning the scattered bits of information into the true interpretation of the universe. It encompasses every sense and every action.

This writing follows the teaching of the all-day transformative conference called *Intentional Wellness*. Learning how to connect the dots in your own being for optimal joy, clarity and wellbeing. Taking control of your own wellness and knowing you hold the key to unlocking the mysteries of the perception of the universe is what *Intentional Wellness* is all about. Live your dream. Create it now.

Chapter I

The Science of Wellness

How miraculous are we? More than we could ever imagine. We are flesh and bone and blood and 100 trillion cells all moving and grooving within the confines of this earthly form we call body. We have come so far as a species in the field of science that we literally seem to be standing on the razor's edge of what reality really is. So much so that we now know there is a reality that is what we see and feel with all of our senses. And then there is 'actuality,' which is how things truly are. We are the wind and the rain; we are the fire and the earth. We carry the trace elements in our body and we are a part of the all that is. And yet there is a vast part of us that remains unknown. That resides within a space smaller than a speck, upon a speck, upon a speck that sits on top of the head of a pin. The very center of spinning space begins at the center of every cell. I believe this is where the secrets of the universe reside. Little bits of spirit, you might say.

It has been a mystery through the ages and only recently have the worlds of science and spirituality started coming together in the quest for the answers of how we connect to the

all and how we are a part of All That Is? Since we are made
up of mostly water and the elements, it makes perfect sense
that we are affected by water and tides, and that the frequency
of water in our bodies may be affected by the frequency of
water everywhere. Water is the element of life's flow.. It rep-
resents our emotions and the movement of water, which gives
off our vibratory rate and so is directly connected to the frequency at which we resonate. And that, my friend, has everything to do with how you experience this lifetime.

The fields of science and wellness are vast indeed. The
amazing discoveries occurring every day are lifting the hope
of humanity. Each and every one of us now knows that what
we put our attention to will manifest. We all now know that
Bioenergetics and neuro-energetics are making their way closer into the mainstream of the medical industry, and that top
scientists and physicians are now validating and encouraging
their patients to try alternative ways of rejuvenating their wellness. Meditation, acutonics, acupuncture, neuro-feedback and
biofeedback, hypnosis and yes, drumming and dancing are now
being considered important components of the wellness of
the whole body.

We are being encouraged to know the components of wellness. How the heart and the brain and every cell are used for
taking in information and transforming it into what we know
as thought and feeling. How we filter and transform the information has everything to do with our being ready, willing and
able to step into our wellness and fulfill our optimal self in
this lifetime. We can work together to create the life of your
dreams. You can create it now.

Quantum Physics and Wellness

From the micro to the macro. From the smallest part to the largest part. This is one of the universal laws of physics. And so we must begin the journey at the smallest part. This gives us a clue to exactly where wellness begins — that everything is energy and energy is information in motion. From the tiniest particle to the vastness of the universe, everything is communicating at all times. We may not see it or hear it, but we know this is true. We cannot see or hear a sound wave but we know it is there. More and more of the population is beginning to awaken to this. Just over the past 10 years, the number of awakening beings have begun to multiply exponentionally.

Can we actually see how this works? Yes! Thanks to our soaring technical advances, we can now experience a wave of information that may be coming from many places.

The new technologically advanced computers can now show you exactly what is going on in your body. The mysteries of our beingness are becoming new discoveries in the world of science and spirituality. More and more we see that we are all one, not separated from the all but a part of it. That our human suffering is an illusion of separation. We can now speak into a machine and have our voice, our sound and vibration analyzed and be given a detailed report of what vitamins, minerals and enzymes we need, our stress levels and where they are coming from, our organ functions and so much more. Ah yes. we seem to be making huge leaps in science and how it applies to our bodies and spirit.

But as sophisticated and wondrous as these machines may seem to be, they cannot hold a candle to the most sophisticated and all-seeing, all-knowing processor in the universe. We carry this integrated and expansive wonder processor within our own physical form, right between our ears. Our own brain is the amazing discovery of this age. How powerful our thoughts are and how we alter the signals to the universe just by our thinking a thought is a discovery that is changing the way we look at all things. Even though we utilize less that 1% of the potential of our brain and mind, our own evolution is pushing us to seek and explore the great adventure. We are the adventure, and as we reach out to fulfill our optimal self, we are activating neurological pathways and turning on switches that have always been within but awaiting this very time in the evolution of our species.

Our evolution is at hand, and we are experiencing a huge leap in global consciousness, not only in ourselves but in every aspect of life on this planet. Intentional Wellness is all about the physics of wellness, and putting together the many pieces of the puzzle to awaken and give new life to the potential that awaits within us.. We are coming full circle as a species, where knowledge turns to wisdom and we know with certainty that we are all connected. Thank you to Dr. Vernon Woolf, Ph.D. for the slides:

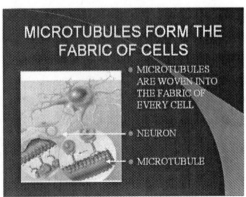

MICROTUBULES FORM THE
FABRIC OF CELLS

• MICROTUBULES
  ARE WOVEN INTO
  THE FABRIC OF
  EVERY CELL

• NEURON

• MICROTUBULE

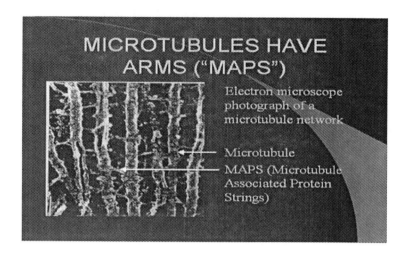

In these two slides, we can actually see how the protein strands connect to each other like a cable wire going through every cell of the body. The neurons travel through the microtubules but they do more than that. Somehow they seem to connect to hyper-space, the grid, non-local space or whatever you choose to call it. It seems to connect us to time and space and has the ability to go beyond time and space.

Chapter 2

Physics of Form

Have you ever watched a school of fish or a flock of birds when they change direction? In a beautiful and instant 'shift,' they appear to all change at the exact same time. I know it looks like an optical illusion but what we witness is communication outside time and space. It actually takes 1/72 of a second. One fish or one bird will receive information of a predator or obstacle, and will change course. As it does, via the quantum field, the thought instantaneously affects the whole school or flock. They are all connected, just as we are.

This connection is what signals the change of all organic matter. Why there are the exact amount of points on a pine cone of same size and age, why the spirals on a shell are perfect. This is called Sacred Geometry and it is the art of matter in the universe. Only in nature do we find perfection and most of nature communicates in non local space and time that is to say it is directly plugged into the universal flow and here is the eye opener, so are you and I.

Our physical form is the housing, the protection for our true self, which is actually energy in motion as all things are energy in motion. Our form is made to take in information and process it. As we do this subconsciously, we are already creating thought and action. Yes it happens in about 1/72 of a second. We are so adaptable and ever changing. But how does this relate to healing? Our being, our form as a human is built to be well, and to see and hear, and live our life in joy. Our cells, our bones and every particle of our being is in a constant cycle of birth, growth, decline, death and re-birth. We continually are rejuvenating ourselves if we allow our natural systems to proceed as planned. We are really built to last. Our mind and brain that process all the information are fully capable of healing themselves if we just have a clue on how this system works and what we can do to help the process of wellness to flourish. It is no accident that our heart is above our center and below the mainframe computer we call "the brain" .It is no accident that our eyes take in the data that the brain translates. Our ears and protective shell that we wear is an amazing design. Every cell in the skin which is the largest organ in the body is like a great big sponge. Feeling the elements and temperature and soft touch or hard touch, even kind touch or not so kind touch all to keep us in our comfort zone as we go on about our day. The entire system is designed for our optimal health and wellbeing and comfort, so how is it so many beings are walking around uncertain of there well being and maybe even wounded in one form or another? That is the question to which this writing will offer you true answers based not only in science but also in the realm of infinite possibilities.

Chapter 3

The Heart

About 8 inches below the top of the chest plate and about 8 inches above the belly button lies a mysterious muscle we call the heart. It is the central pump that keeps all systems going. It communicates with every cell and gives instructions to the brain. I feel a deeper look is warranted when it comes to the heart. It is also an area from which a large energy field can now be measured. The picture below was shown at a conference with Howard Martin who is a pioneer in the field of "Heart Math." It was amazing as he explained the pattern of energy that emanates from the heart. As you can see, it resembles a figure 8, a never-ending circle folded in on itself. Like a strand

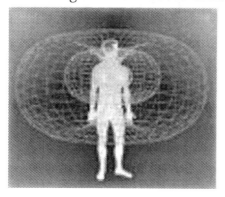

of DNA the energy pulses out into atheric space. This is the electromagnetic field of the heart, the energy signature that may not be seen but is ever present. It is the pattern of our life force, beautiful and fragile as we all are.

Some years ago while at a Prophets' Conference Howard Martin also unveiled an amazing discovery. While talking about the energy signature of the heart he also mentioned that for many years, it has been thought that our brain is the hub, the system that runs our Reality. It's all in the mind, right? Recently, however, it was discovered that there are more signals that go from the heart to the brain than from the brain to the heart. What an amazing discovery. The implications are that it is the heart that is the hub. The heart and the brain work together to transform the Information into what we know as thought and feeling. There are many scientists that will tell you that the brain is the hub, the all seeing all knowing component of this human form. There is at this time no definitive answer. It is my belief that it is a symbiotic relationship. That the brain and the heart work together in harmony bringing us a moment to moment up date on the world and everything around us at any given time.

The heart is the giver of life, the central pump that in its rhythmic pulsing moves all the magic ingredients through our body such as blood and oxygen, cells that heal and protect our very being. The heart also is sending signals to every cell and organ, keeping a constant monitor on who needs what. If you need oxygen, you will take a breath; if you need to get rid of an invading germ or particle, you will sneeze; our heart speaks to us every moment of every day. But who is listening?

When you have heartburn, do you go within and ask, "What has caused this?" Do you heed the clues and communication you receive from your heart? In all relationships, communication is key to keeping it healthy, so why do we stop when it comes to our own body? Back in the 80's I was listening to John Bradshaw, a pioneer in the field of emotional intelligence. He said "My heat tried to tell me in so many ways, it tried to let me know but I wasn't listening. It finally got so mad that it attacked me! I had a heart attack and that finally got my attention" I never forgot those words and find the concept to be true and valid. So how do we communicate with our body?

If you lie quietly for a few moments and close your eyes, scan your own body and listen to how and what it is saying. Some people believe there are only so many beats in any given heart and when that count runs out, so do you. I disagree and think it is that limiting thought and belief system that creates the intention of death from a very young age. It is this belief system that causes the heart to stop prematurely. The intention and belief in death create the unconscious behavior and sees death as the goal and complies. I believe we were made to be here for a very long time, to learn and discover our inner connection to our heart , our soul and all of the universe. To be at one with our self and live from the heart. You know when you are putting something into your body that is harmful to your heart, you get a voice message that says "This is really bad for me" or "This will be the last one" or I know I must change my ways. That my friend is your body talking to you making an effort to guide you. We do not always listen but our bodies do always give us an opportunity to choose what is in the best interest of our self.

What we put into our bodies is vitally important to the health of our heart but perhaps even more important is what and how we think. This may have more profound effects on our precious heart. Our intention has a direct link to how our heart will respond to any and all situations.

At the seed of every thought, our heart takes the information and sends it to the brain and every cell of the entire body so the chemistry changes, It is a constant flow of change in every moment.

Those Sayings Really Do Have a Meaning

Over the years there have been many sayings about the heart and most of them actually have a foundation. When someone says, "It's the heart of the matter," we know exactly what that means. That it is the center, the core. It is the ticking life-maker that brings us to life in this realm.

When someone says, "Have a heart," we all know this means to have compassion, to reach into our hearts and come forth with kindness and understanding.

When we say, "Don't break my heart," everyone knows this means our heart is so precious and how our heart is feeling affects every aspect of every system in our body, mind and spirit.

The heart seems to reach beyond all time and reason. It has the capacity to bring us to the heights of ecstasy and then dive to the depths of despair and back again.

It has long been thought that the brain connects to the universal grid. It has only been a handful of years since the discovery was made that it is indeed the heart that connects us, not only to the grid but also to spirit and the soul as well. We can feel when we are close to spirit and all feelings emote from the heart.

On our journey to Intentional Wellness, it is the heart we will be communicating with. It is the true feelings that we need to explore and unravel the 'pockets of opportunity.' It is the heart that will heal the body, mind and spirit.

Now would be a great time to honor and embrace your beautiful heart. Thank your heart and be grateful for each and every glorious day.

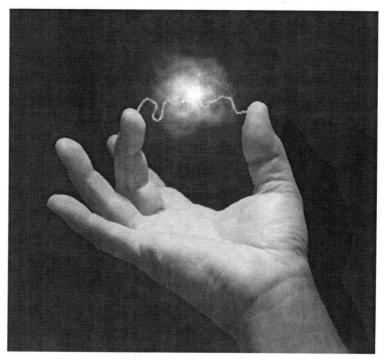

The Body Electric

I love this picture. It shows how we are electrical in nature. Our bodies are governed by the current, the life force that is contained within. The heart has a constant current. So do you think that the current is affected by the intention and the perspective from which we view life? An interesting question and yes, I believe this current is connected directly to the grid and also to our unconscious mind. So how important is it that we begin to synchronize the conscious and unconscious mind? There is unlimited electrical current moving through the universe. Just by being aware of this fact, you have started the process of unfolding the awareness that may boost your life force. We are the body electric.

Chapter 4

Right Brain, Left Brain

Throughout history the brain has been a subject of scientific study and fascination. I would like to share a few quotes with you as we see the diversity of thought that has been explored.

"The greatest discovery of my generation is that man can alter his life simply by altering his attitude of mind."

— *William James (1842-1910)*

"And of course, the brain is not responsible for any of the sensations at all. The correct view is that the seat and source of sensation is the region of the heart."

— *Aristotle*

"I never came upon any of my discoveries through the process of rational thinking."

— *Albert Einstein*

"In proportion to our body mass, our brain is three times as large as that of our nearest relatives. This huge organ is dangerous and painful to give birth to, expensive to build and, in a resting human, uses about 20 per cent of the body's energy even though it is just 2 per cent of the body's weight. There must be some reason for all this evolutionary expense."

— *Susan Blakemore (from "Me, Myself, I,"* New Scientist, *March 13, 1999*

"The brain gives the heart its sight. The heart gives the brain its vision."

— *Kall*

"Our brain, like a nurturing mother will reason and reach for logic and understanding while simotainously being the fierce warrior that protects and defends its precious child and that precious child is the beating heart that lives within us all."

— *Sheila Z Stirling*

"Logic will get you from A to B. Imagination will take you everywhere."

— *Albert Einstein*

The brain is one of the last and most mysterious frontiers yet to be figured out. We know that as humans we are using a very small portion of what we are sent here with. It is possible that as we explore consciousness and the expanding of one's imagination that we may very well be activating and awakening more and more connecters. Below are some explanations as I feel it is so important for us to grasp the functions and the feeling of the brain and the heart before getting into the mechanics of cellular re-patterning. The ORT technique is a form of cellular re-patterning, as we will be discussing in chapter 23.

The Wikipedia explains the lateralization of brain function like this: "The human brain is separated by a longitudinal fissure, separating the brain into two distinct cerebral hemispheres connected by the corpus callosum. The two sides of the brain are similar in appearance, and every structure in each hemisphere is generally mirrored on the other side. Despite these strong similarities, the functions of each cortical hemisphere are different, being lateralized, that is, located in the right or left side of the brain. These ideas need to be treated carefully because the popular lateralizations are often distributed across both sides. However, there is some division of mental processing. Probably most fundamental to brain lateralization is the fact that the lateral sulcus is generally longer in the left hemisphere than in the right hemisphere. Researchers have been investigating to what extent areas of the brain are specialized for certain functions. If a specific region of the brain is injured or destroyed, their functions can sometimes be recovered by neighboring brain regions – even opposite hemispheres. This depends more on the age and the damage occurred than anything else.

"It is important to note that, while functions are indeed lateralized, these lateralizations are trends and do not apply to every person in every case."

Some of the characteristics of the left-brain are:

- Rational
- Logical
- Sequential
- Safe
- Practical
- Present and past
- Facts rule
- Analytical
- Objective

Some of the characteristics of the right brain are:

- Random
- Intuitive
- Holistic
- Uses feeling
- Synthesizing
- Subjective
- Looks at wholes
- Risk-taking
- Present and future
- Imagination rules.

It is said that the right brain houses most of the creative connectors; that is to say, if you are interested in art, nature and beauty, it is mostly the right brain activity that sends the messages and also connects to the emotion. The amygdule is the feeling part of the brain, the right brain. The neo-cortex is the thinking part of the brain, the left brain. For all the accountants, computer programmers and those who seek logic in every moment, it is safe to say you are more comfortable in your left brain. For many, as life pushes your limits, you become more and more comfortable in the left side or logical side of the brain because it keeps you from feeling the emotion of a feeling.

This all sounds great until you realize that the feeling is always there, waiting for a time when you will embrace that which brings you emotional discomfort, and start feeling again. We all know. "You can't heal what you can't feel."

We are like a giant recording machine, in that every sense, every event, every word and every thought is recorded and held in the cells. Like a massive filing cabinet, we remember and store every moment of our life.

Some scientists say that the brain is not the mind. That the brain is the non-physical, the feeling and experiential part of the equation and the mind is the place where memory is stored. There have been documented cases where a person with very small amount of brain matter is getting A's and B's in school. Something is going on. The mind takes over when the brain is not available.

I bring this up because it is important to know it does not matter if you think you are smart or not smart. It does not matter if your grades could have been better in school. What matters is that you are open enough to realize you are on the brink of a wonderful change, a leap in your evolution.

An Amazing Discovery

I would like to share with you some information about what is called a neuro-feedback machine. Many new machines are making great advancements in the field of mind/brain training or balancing. In my case, I did the neuro-feedback for head trauma injuries, but this type of information and therapy is good for anyone who wants to know where and how their brain is functioning. During my recovery, the neuro-feedback machine was considered a new technology, and only a few treatments helped me more than anything. I was hooked up to a machine much like an EEG, with electrodes placed strategically on my head to show the signals from my brain. Once the machine was turned on, it showed the alpha, beta, theta and

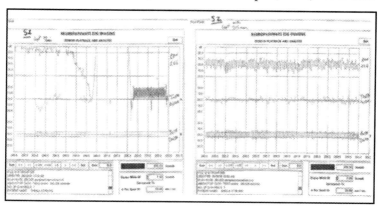

delta brain waves on a monitor. My job was to just sit and watch the monitor. The amazing part was that all I had to do was stare at the screen, and my eyes would see my brain waves malfunctioning and my brain began to fix itself based on what my eyes were seeing. It was proof positive that our human form is fully capable and awaiting instructions to fulfill our optimal wellness. Whether you fell off your bike at the age of 7, broke your leg at the age of 10, or went through a very difficult and emotional divorce or loss, these neuro-feedback machines tell you immediately how your brain is functioning. It is important to note that the way we learn as humans is through trauma and events that push us to our limits. When we are ready, a catalyst will show up in our life, intended for our growth and transformation.

The chart on a previous page is a raw EEG of the left side of my head. As you can see, the left side is well, shall we say, out there. As you can see, alpha, beta, theta and delta brain-waves are way out of normal range. On the right side of the chart is where I put headphones on with *Sounds of the Soul* playing. To everyone's amazement, it seems the sounds have a normalizing effect on all the brainwaves associated with this EEG.

The prospects of this, I must say, are more than promising and you will see this chart in other places in this book.

Chapter 5

Perception

We are in a time and place of boundryless possibilities
— Sheila Z

Perception is defined as: "An act or result of perceiving," "awareness of environment through physical sensation," and "ability to perceive." I would like to add to this. Perception is what happens when all the cells and all the views and all the past and present, and perhaps the future, come together in a nanosecond and in that moment, all the input we have had up to that moment defines what our perception will be in that same moment. It is a wondrous feat of all the systems working together to allow us to have a single thought and a single perspective. When we feel love, it is this mechanism at work. Also when we feel hurt.

No two people will have the exact same perception of anything. Each one of us has a long history of thoughts, feelings and experiences that define how we perceive.

In the end, our life is our perception of life. Even the perception of 'the end' is a perception because the truth is, nothing really ends, it just transforms. Scientifically speaking, that is a fact. When we say, "Dust to dust." we mean that literally. Our atoms have been the same atoms that have been in this time and space since the beginning of this time and space. How we perceive our world and act or react will determine the level of happiness, joy and fulfillment we receive in our life. Our life is our perception of our life.

I'd like to tell a little story about perception.

A number of years ago a dear friend of mine, actually a spiritual mentor, from Hawaii came to visit. Her name was Dawna Su and she was known as the great mother, the nurturer on the Island of Kauai. She was a wonderful woman who had developed many of her psychic and spiritual gifts and made her living giving soul readings to people all over the world. At one point in her readings, she would pull out a deck of round cards. They were a beautiful lavender in color and when you turned them over, they would give you words of wisdom, like a deck of oracle cards. I always felt good about those cards and really wanted a deck of my own. I had looked in all the New Age and book stores I could find when I would travel to other cities to see if they had this deck, but to no avail. On this particular visit, we went into a New Age store and I felt a dark presence there. I didn't frequent the store myself, nor did I buy things there as I was privy to some inside unethical behavior on the part of the owners. However, Dawna Su wanted to go there and so off we went.

As we walked through the store, the smell of incense was thick, and Dawna Su loved to touch everything in the store. There were bells and books and crystals and clothes. Brooms hung from the ceiling and large statues stood at every corner of the store. Along the entire back wall of the store was a large glass case. As I looked in the glass case, I could hardly believe my eyes …. there on the third shelf down, lying on a beautiful purple velvet bag, was a deck of the round lavender oracle cards. I called Dawna Su over and said, "I cannot buy these cards from this store. I don't feel right about it."

From my perspective, I would be doing the right thing by not buying this deck of cards from this particular store even though I had searched for them for over a year. As I was telling Dawna Su a story of why I felt I could not purchase these cards and was getting ready to walk away, she took hold of my arm, looked straight into my eyes, and what she said next shifted my entire perception of the situation.. She said, *"My dear, this is a rescue mission!* You *must* buy these cards because this is a rescue mission!"

In that moment, my perception shifted and I could see the wisdom of her words. I bought the deck and felt good in my heart for rescuing these cards of light. It's all a matter of perception.

Our perception of ourselves and the world around us has everything to do with the way our reality unfolds.

Chapter 6

Sound, Vibration and Frequency

Everything is information in motion
— Dr. Steven Hawkins *The Universe in a Nut Shell*

The universe was draped in silence, then the silence was broken by sound. The waves swept across the galaxy in a silent symphony, heard only by the elements and the vast space of the cosmos. And so began our world of frequencies, vibrations and sound. Everything carries its own unique frequency. Every plant, every flower, every tree and insect, birds, rocks, water, and yes, people. Everything is made of sound, light, and vibration. The vehicle is energy.

Everything is energy, and energy is information in motion. We are all connected to the universe by the unified field. This information, energy and frequencies are moving continually. Everything the eye can see, although it looks to be a stable form, is really sound and vibration.

Recently, many quantum physicists such as Dr. Vernon Woolf are proving the theories that we are, in fact, holographic. To be holographic is to know that every cell carries the pattern of every other cell. The cells are in constant communication and so when someone says, "The only way to truly heal is on a cellular level," we see that it may take a specific technique to reach not only one cell but also all 100 trillion cells. This must happen from the space that is non-local and yet will happen in an instant. We do not have, nor do we want, control. It is the act of letting go and embracing the true feeling that releases the trauma.

So what does this mean to our own wellness? When our body and our organs and our cells are working in harmony – that beautiful silent symphony that is sound and vibration – everything is in order. When you have something in the body that is not in harmony, some people call it dis-ease.

I believe, in the not too distant future, it is harmonic resonance and frequencies that will realign the balance of the organs or tissues, and you will experience wellness once again. So when we speak of sound and frequencies as a healing modality, it is a modality that speaks to every cell in the body. Certain tones, certain notes, promote wellness. You know when you hear them. Your body knows when you hear them. Have you ever listened to a piece of music that just makes you want to sit down, close your eyes, and listen? And as a contrast, have you also heard music that makes you feel upset or at ill ease, and you just want to shut it off? If you allow the body to express itself, the body will always tell you which music is aligned to your soul and which music is not.

Music is called the universal language. Sound and vibration is a common thread that weaves its way through the very fabric of all life as we know it.

So how do we use sound to heal ourselves? Let's talk about meditation for a while. It is a well known fact that meditation has been used as a healing modality for thousands of years. In every religion, every spiritual teaching, there is a form of meditation. It is in these quiet places that we open the doorway for true healing. I like to say meditation is the pathway to visualization, and visualization is the pathway to wellness.

When you sit quietly, begin to breathe, breathing in the tones of healing music, you allow yourself to travel inward to the deepest part of your being. Begin to feel yourself shifting. If you have a guide, as in guided meditation, sometimes it makes this traveling easier. If you have a pre-set idea of what kind of visualizations will work for you, the visualizations become stronger and stronger as you do them more and more.

Just as aligning the conscious and the subconscious will begin to transform the information that flows within every cell; using sound and vibration to reach the core of your being is a key element in becoming your own healer.

We already know that sound has a profound effect on the body, including the blood cells. This is not new. Through the works of Simon Heather and the research done, we can see how multi-dimensional music and sound have a profound effect on the blood cells. Jonathon Goldman said, "We are a wind instrument," and I say, " every cell, all 100 trillion of them, are vibrating and resonating at specific frequencies." This brings us to actuality and life as we know it in this realm.

As you may know, since the moment of the Blessing in the form of an auto accident in 1999, I have had "tinitasis" a ringing in both ears. On paper, it shows this has affected my hearing; in reality I hear very well. On a trip to the mountains I had an awesome experience, a miracle for me for sure, where opening to the sounds of nature caused me a few moments peace from the ringing. The sound waves coming from the water synchronized with the sound waves of the ringing and I experienced silence. It was so amazing for me that I sat down and wrote a small poem about it and I would like to share it with you.

Sounds of Silence

In the sound of the shoreline I find silence.

The lake is crystal clear this early summer morning.

The smooth sheet-like patches on the water reflect like giant mirrors.

Dark blue, turquoise and crystal clear as far as the eye can see.

The surging waves lap at the shoreline and in that glorious sound I find silence.

The vastness is breathtaking.

Again and again and again the water surrounds my feet inviting me in.

As I breathe in the clean mountain air, I see mother-nature in all of her splendor,

offering me the kinship of this ancient place.

Infusing me with healing minerals from a time before time.

I am so grateful to be standing here right now in this moment.

For in the sounds of the shoreline I find silence.

In the surging waves lapping at my feet there is peace.

Finally silence, finally peace.

— sheila z

The Technology of Frequency

In 1992, Bruce Taino of Taino Technology, an independent division of Eastern State University in Cheny, Washington, built the first frequency monitor in the world. Taino determined that the average frequency of a healthy human body during the day time is 62 – 68 Hz. When the frequency drops, the immune system is compromised. If the frequency drops to 58 Hz, cold and flu symptoms appear; at 55 Hz, diseases like Candida take hold; at 52 Hz, Epstein Bar and at 42 Hz, Cancer. Taino's machine was certified as 100 percent accurate and is currently being used in the agricultural field today. According to Dr. Royal R. Rife, every disease has a frequency. He has found that certain frequencies can prevent the development of disease and that others would destroy diseases. Substances of higher frequency will destroy diseases of lower frequency.

It is a proven fact that sound moves matter. In the awareness of just that, we know with certainty that sound has a profound effect on the body and all matter in the universe.

On my channeled CD *Sounds of the Soul*, this multidimensional music seems to have the perfect resonance to balance and normalize brain waves as seen in the chart below.

This is actually a neuro-feedback graph that measures Alpha, Beta, Theta, and Delta brain waves. As you can see, and as we talked about in Chapter 4, the brain waves that are without the music are way outside normal range in every aspect. The consistency of the brain wave is nonexistent on the left side of the graph. And when *Sounds of the Soul* is played through headphones, all the brain waves go into balance and into nor-

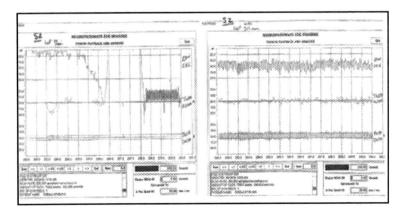

mal range. This is significant and tangible proof of how sound and vibration affect the mind, body and spirit.

Chapter 7

How the Past Defines the Future

So you come into the world a precious, angelic being. You look up at the faces of your source figures, that is to say your mother or father, or even a sister or brother, grandparents etc., – the family that welcomes you into the world. If you see smiles most of the time, and most babies do see smiles most of the time, you will learn to smile. Most of our expressions come from what we saw during the first year of our journey in this world. If you have ever met someone who does not show a lot of facial expression, chances are that if you met their family, you would find that same trait.

So much of who we become is a direct result of the environmental factors, that is, our surroundings and the behaviors of the people who were in our family circle. This goes for everyone, including you if you were an orphan or adopted. When you look into the eyes of a young baby and coo and smile, you are teaching that child how to coo and smile. When you hold a young child in your arms and rock him or her to sleep, he is learning trust and safety and loving kindness. And here is the astonishing thing – a good percentage of what a child will pick up will be on a subconscious level. That is why they say so many traits can be multi-generational.

As an example, I was born into a loving family where neither my mom or dad drank or smoked. (Well, my dad would have a shot of whisky every night but he made it very clear that his doctor said it was good for his heart.) My parents were both older than most. My mom was in her mid-forties when I was born and my father was 12 years her senior so that would make him in his late fifties. Poor fellow. Anyway, when I was born, my father already had a heart condition and, as we know, sometimes a flashy temper can be a side-effect of high blood pressure or a heart condition. So growing up I would witness outbreaks when my dad would raise his voice and sometimes say things he did not really mean. But, because he was a source figure for me, I saw his actions as love. I knew he loved me and I just overlooked some of his anger, as we all did. The funny thing is, I married someone who had the same trait as my father. Unknowingly and subconsciously, I still viewed this as love.

This is how what we call 'patterns' are born.

As we hear, see, think and smell, our cells begin to adapt to the environment in which we spend our time. Even at a young age and unknowingly, our thoughts do become things. We are constantly adapting and doing whatever it takes to fit into the place we are standing, which in most cases means into our family. So, one child might take on the role of caretaker and another might take on the roll of jester, knowing that helping people to laugh is a good thing. There are 'rebels' and 'scape-goats,' and many more 'labels.'

The bottom line is that we inherently do what we must to survive and thrive. So the behaviors and the things we do as children follow us into adulthood, silently affecting our perception, actions and reactions.

Every moment, we are taking in data and storing the information in our cells. It is well-known that an adult screaming at a child under the age of 4 will traumatize the young child and change the brain chemistry of that child forever. This is shocking if we think back about how many times we were yelled at, or for that matter, how many times we have yelled at our own children.

When we are unable to deal with a situation, our body stores this information in the cells. I call them "Pockets of Opportunity," and each one alters our perception of the world around us ever so slightly. As a result, how we act and react are changed and patterns are born.

It would be wonderful if there were classes that, when you turned 18, became mandatory because at that age, the 'patterns' would still be easier to unwind. However, since that does not happen, these 'files' are stored in the cells of the body and, as we go through life, they pop up as a reminder that this would be a good time to deal with what I call the file or pocket of opportunity. As a rule, most people view these as times of loss or sorrow, along with emotions such as anger, jealousy and resentment.

The secret is: "You cannot heal what you cannot feel." The key element to releasing these old files is getting back to the feeling of it, pinpointing the emotion, and recognizing it. You cannot change something until you know it is there.

We will be discussing the technique for embracing and releasing these pockets in Chapter 23.

Chapter 8

Emotional Baggage

Okay, let's talk about emotional baggage. What is baggage? It implies that this "stuff" is "extra, has no use and no value and that: "Baggage is something we must get rid of to be healthy, wealthy and wise." Right? Wrong! I have a very different view and here it is:

It is true we are affected by every moment and every event. Our human form is one of taking in and receiving information – all information – translating and transforming this information into behaviors and beliefs, actions and re-actions to the input, or the data we process. Before you go throwing this information away, know that it is this information that has guided and formed you into the magnificent being you are today. It is this information that holds the keys to unlocking the door to our fulfilled and optimal self.

From the time we came through the tunnel at the edge of the womb, and maybe even before, we started this journey of taking in information and translating it and growing from it. Continual change is the name of the process and it is as much apart of us as breathing.

When we are young and forming our perspectives of this life and this world, we have limited "local" ability to process the information. There are events we cannot decipher and so this information is stored in the vast space we call the self. This information is always flowing and always meant for our greatest knowing, always intended for our highest good.

There is always a blessing and a universal invitation for growth and wisdom. We store un-deciphered information in files. As we pile file upon file upon file, we fall behind in the intended processing and transformation. This is the stuff most people refer to as baggage.

I call them "Pockets of Opportunity" – bits of information that have been stored that we can access, process and transform. This gives us the opportunity to know the blessing and receive the growth and wisdom from it.

First of all, these "Pockets of Opportunity" or "POO" are apart of our neuro network. They are stored in every cell and every feeling, so you really could not throw it away even if you tried.

Some of these pockets get worked out on their own as we journey through this life. When you have an 'Ah ha,' moment or sudden shift in understanding, more than likely a 'POO' was embraced, transformed and released. This is a natural event and wonderful when it happens that way.

There are those files and pockets that will remain until we seek them out. Go back to the moment, take the information into your heart, and allow your light to shine on it – your light of understanding, compassion, gratitude, and love. We are built for this. Our bodies are made for this. When you do this, the blessing will be revealed. The "charge" will be released, your heart will open, and tears of gratitude will flow. When you embrace this, the transformation will occur. As this information is revealed in its entirety, every cell in your body will respond. There will be a shift in your perception and this sometimes very subtle shift will ripple through every cell and outward into the universe. Another piece of the puzzle will have been put in place. And, of course, the more pieces of the puzzle we put in place, the clearer the picture becomes. How we love those moments of clarity and certainty.

You must know that sometimes, when we open a Pocket of Opportunity, it may be a huge awakening and clearing with a river of tears. The shift may be profound and that is wonderful, indeed. As we go through these files, these pockets, our cells are re-patterning to the new lighter frequency. Each and every cell releases its piece of the file. This is a very healthy endeavor, and a way we can honor ourselves and honor all that we have come through. It honors the whole self, the precious being we came in as. By doing this work, we honor our own growth and incredible full potential. It is another beautiful crystal on the path to total wellness. It is your birthright and one of the reasons we came to this planet at this time.

Chapter 9

Feeling and Emotion

You may be saying to yourself at this very minute, "Feelings and emotions are the same thing, right?"

Well that would be one perspective, but in the world of actuality that would be not correct. Just as perception and windows are similar but not the same because they differ in origin, feelings come from the heart. We may feel happy or sad or grateful or full of loss. It is coming directly from our inner self and is a true expression of the heart. Feeling implies it is an 'inside job'; feeling is the place we want to go to be able to embrace and release the 'pockets of opportunity.' Only with true feeling can this be accomplished.

No one can really make us feel a certain way. It comes down to our own perspective that feeds into the heart and a feeling is born. Be it love, sorrow it stems from our perspective of a given situation.

Emotion tends to be connected to the ego, to the exterior personality. An overlay if you will on a feeling. You may say "Oh he or she makes me angry". The truth is the emotion of anger is a perception of the wearer. An expectation unfulfilled, we react as if some one else has done something to us when in fact it is our own illusion that has us in a reaction. When the ego is bruised, hurt, or pushed in any way, we get emotional. It feels almost like a feeling but it is so very different. Sometimes emotion comes up and we wonder, "Where did that com from?" The answer is usually that long ago, we were unable to deal or cope with a situation, so it was stored in a file, a pocket! And now someone has come into your world, sent by the universe to let you know you are now ready and able to deal with it. People, places, and things will be brought into your world when the time is right. The opportune moment! The challenge is that most people do not see the opportunity and react with emotion. So guess what? The opportunity will keep on coming up until you finally get it and deal with it.

The next time you think someone has made you mad or sad, stop, close your eyes, take a deep breath and ask where this feeling is really coming from. Just breath, open your heart and mind, and the answer will come. You will then open the door to the opportunity to explore, embrace and re-pattern the event, which honors it and allows it to be released. The universe just works that way.

Our feelings are the culmination of the cellular information that rushes through our system. The information on a cellular level will give the impulses to the heart and create joy and sorrow, and create an open heart or a closed heart. Our feelings come from the deepest part of our being and there are no wrong feelings. No two feelings are the same. Feelings create our deepest form of desires and our transformations.

Emotions are our own reaction to our feelings, and can be affected by our ego and outside forces. Emotions are more closely related to *reactions*, while feelings are more closely related to *actions*. We all have feelings and emotions. How we show up and how we act or react to a given feeling or emotion is a benchmark for where we are in our own conscious and spiritual evolution.

Chapter 10

Perception & Windows

In Chapter 5, we discussed perception, so how does a "window" differ from perception? Just as emotion is an overlay on feelings (as we discussed in the previous chapter), so a window is an overlay on our perception. Perception is the accumulation of all available data that has been stored. A window is how we look outward into the world, like an overlay on the perception.

The data is in every cell and the body interprets this information and we see from our very own and specific window. No two people look from the same window. How special and wonderful to find a person or many people that have a similar view. Not the same view bit similar. Have you ever seen or heard something and told someone about it. Then you hear back from someone else what you had said and it is so different that you could hardly recognize it as what you had originally said. Now, some people may think there is some malicious gossiping going on but, most of the time, each person really does hear their own interpretation of what was said, so every time the story is retold, it is altered slightly.

If we remember that each person has his or her own window, and therefore a unique view of how the world is supposed to be, then we realize that every person has the right to his or her own window. Then, we begin to understand that it is our *own* judgment on things and our *own* perception that can cause discomfort. It's a given that when we look out our own window, we see things from our own view. It takes a little more effort to know and to respect the fact that *every* person is doing exactly the same thing. When we honor and respect the windows of other people, our own life becomes enriched exponentially.

So the next time someone tells you that you live in a dream world or see the world through rose-colored glasses, just say, "Thank you," and know that they are seeing you through their own window and that it's their own perception that is making the judgment. It has little to do with what you may or may not be doing in your life, for only you know the windows you peer out from.

Chapter II

Your Inner Voice

Oh yes, that wonderful inner voice that sometimes can build us up or tear us down. We all have one, an inner voice and an outer voice. Our conscious mind is our outer voice. It lies on the surface and seemingly expresses what it is we want, we feel, we have, or have not in that moment. All of the thoughts that lie in the conscious mind may seem to lie in the realm of reality but that is an illusion. It is the subconscious mind that lives in the realm of actuality. It is the synchronization of the conscious and subconscious with the certainty of intention that can be the driving force of wellness. Let's explore this a little more deeply.

Have you ever experienced a situation where somebody asked you how you felt and outwardly you said, "I'm feeling great," while at the very same time, your inner voice is saying, "I really don't feel well at all. My knee hurts. I have a pain in my back, and something going on in my head."

Has it ever happened to you? Or have you ever been introduced to somebody and you say, "Hi, how are you doing? Very nice to meet you." At the same time, inside a critical voice may be saying, "Wow what was she thinking with the color of her hair," or, "That's the ugliest sweater I've ever seen."

A third example of this, and the one I feel is the most important to pay attention to, comes if you ever taken on a job or a new position, or you're doing something in life that may seem new to you, and somebody says to you, "You're doing a great job," or, "Hey, that's really neat." On the outside, you're saying, "Thank you, isn't this wonderful," but on the inside, you're feeling doubtful and self critical, maybe hearing something similar to, "Who do you think you are?" or, "What do you think you're doing?"

If this sounds familiar to you, it's okay for you're not alone. It is this inner voice that can make our best intentions seem very far away and can keep our Intentional Wellness just out of our reach. It is the subconscious that is really running the show. The conscious mind tends to be more related to the ego or the outer self, whereas the subconscious tends to be more related to the heart and your true feelings.

Synchronizing the inner voice and the outer voice is an important key to your living the life you desire. It is a skill that may indeed be inherent but somehow for most, forgotten long ago. The good news is this skill can be learned just like any other skill. Let's begin with the conscious mind. The conscious mind, sees hears, takes in data from all the senses. The conscious mind knows when something feels good or doesn't feel good. Most people simply ignore the subconscious mind as random chatter that seems to be nagging and biting on the heels of emotion. The subconscious mind has a stronger inherent connection to what is really going on at a cellular level. The subconscious mind has also been affected by the information we have experienced from our birth and perhaps even before. Similar to what was stated in Chapter 9 about how our past defines our future, as a small child our source figures – your mother, father, brother, sister, any adult who may have had an influence on your life when you were very young – programmed our subconscious. How many of us heard, "Stop, don't do that," Or, "Stop, you can't do that," or maybe. "Your big brother can do that but you can't"?

Knowing that our cells record every moment of everything that happens in our life, unless we do something to go back and reset or release or embrace these thoughts we are destined to play them over and over throughout our life. When the thought is transformed, it is chemically released within all 100 trillion cells of the body. This is why it is so important to synchronize the subconscious and conscious mind to be one with who you truly are. Every single being comes in with all of the information needed to have a fulfilling life, a life of wellness, prosperity, and happiness. And if you're thinking to yourself right now, after reading those words: *Well I don't think that means me, because I've had too many things happen in my life then,* this is exactly for you. It may feel as if the conscious mind is running the show and I know I'm repeating myself, but as we begin to hear and recognize more of what our subconscious voice is saying, we begin to realize it is that *inner* voice that is creating our reality.

So what can we do?

One of the techniques used in synchronizing the conscious and subconscious is meditation and visualization. Meditation is the pathway that takes us to visualization and visualization is the pathway to transformation. As an exercise, each day take a moment and find your center place of peace and give your subconscious an affirmation that will help to uplift your inner voice.

Even if you don't believe it at first, if you say it enough, write it enough, think it enough, the cells of the body will begin to change and transform into what that thought form is.

For example, sit down somewhere quiet, take a few breaths, and listen to the inner chatter.. It may be positive, negative or somewhere in between. Think about something you'd like to tell yourself. Think about something that would help this inner part of you to understand what a beautiful and precious being you are. If you're going into a new position and you have doubts about it, you might say, over and over, to yourself, "I am ready, willing and able to do this new job. I am the perfect person to fulfill this job. I am capable of fulfilling all that is asked of me, and I know with certainty that this job will be a wonderful, uplifting experience in my life."

Visualize in your mind what that looks like. See yourself happy, fulfilled and doing this new position with the greatest of ease. If you do this every day, at least once a day, within a short while, you may see things change for the better, not only in that position, but in all aspects of your life. In this way, you can start to train the inner voice to become more in alignment with who you truly are. If you have a doubt, embrace it. Love it and begin to understand where it came from. The moment your subconscious understands where this doubt came from completely, it will be released. That is to say, this may not happen in an hour or a day or a week, but it can. Most transformations happen in an instant. Getting to that moment may take a little time.

Chapter 12

Thoughts Are Things

(Excerpt from Longevity through Spiritual Wellness by Sheila Z Stirling)

As we know, thought and the spoken word come forth into this world like millions of vibrations pushing through the etheric field. So, as a young girl wakes up in California with hope and promise in her heart, and a deep desire to promote peace and tolerance her voice, her intent rings out as if there is no space or time between her and the young girl who wakes up in New York or Chicago and feels for the first time … "Something is different! I will no longer go with the crowd. I believe in peace and in love and a better way. And I am ready to stand up for what I am feeling in my heart."

Do we know with certainty that these two young girls are connected? Or is it just coincidence? Quantum Physics shows us that, in the unified field, everything is connected. So, as a new day dawns across this nation, it is birthed in every corner of the globe. In non-local connection, there is no space and time.

Thoughts really are things. The energy that is in movement through out the brain and the neuro-chemistry taking place within the cells can be measured. As the information makes its way through the miles and miles of pathways, it is alive with information that we translate and transform into thought and then into action or into a form of action we choose to share the information with. The thought itself creates the neuro-chemicals that then connect through the unified field to every cell in the body and you guessed it! It takes only 1/72 of a second to do this enormous feat. Our thoughts are at the core of every movement, every belief and every moment of life. We are now beginning to realize that to choose the good thoughts may be the way to open to the universe in a whole new and more effective way.

It feels to me as if every day the thoughts are manifesting into things much more quickly. How does it feel to you? Is it my perception or is it that at this time in the universe the energies are really strong and transformative? As our frequencies heighten, so shall the manifesting heighten. When we take or make the time to really be specific about what we would like to see in a positive way, it allows the universe to set the wheels in motion. Remember, we are always manifesting our thoughts.

Well, what if we have bad thoughts?

There is no question that we are a balanced being and that there is a negative thought perhaps rolling around unseen and unspoken. And that is the perfect place for that. It is of the utmost importance that we realize that all thought is just that. If we have a thought that seems dark or not something we would like to see for ourselves, that thought is valid nonetheless and so needs to be embraced and once again explored for where its origin is. Do not give the negative thought any energy and it will subside. When we embrace it and understand where it came from, it will unwind itself and be gone. The more we dwell on, "Oh NO, I have bad thoughts!" the more they will manifest. With all the thousands of TV clips that flash in front of our eyes each day, we are keenly aware of some of the darker aspects of what may be going on in the world. Just know, all is in divine balance and keep your heart on seeing the good and the transformation, and know that without the darkness, we would not see the light. We have free will and the choice to bring to the forefront whatever thoughts we desire to manifest. We choose the good thoughts and those thoughts that will uplift not only *our* consciousness but also the consciousness of the whole world. It is happening as you're reading these words. And if that statement brought a smile to your face, then know for sure, you are part of the great transformation going on right here, right now. We choose the good thoughts because we have the choice.

Our energy and thoughts of hope, happiness, love and laughter are helping to illuminate and raise the frequency of the world. Remembering that energy is energy, we really begin to see and get it that our own inner voice and our thoughts and intention have an astounding effect on consciousness everywhere and yes, even the state of well-being for mother earth herself. Yes, thoughts are things and our thoughts and intention can move mountains.

Chapter 13

The Art of Manifesting

The synchronization of the conscious and unconscious mind

We all know manifesting seems to be the current buzzword. Manifesting is not new; it has been around since the beginning of time. We are all manifesting all the time. That means every single one of us is manifesting in every single moment. Unknowingly, we play a major role in how our life unfolds. The real difference now is that we have matured enough as a species to realize that we really do play a role in how our life and our world unfolds. Before now, we created our reality unknowingly, but now we know our thoughts and attitudes are a precursor and play a big role in our unfolding world.

Where do we go from here? Yes, what you focus on will manifest. What you think about will come to be. So why is it everything in your life isn't perfect? The answer lies in the subconscious as talked about in Chapter 11.

It starts with the conscious mind. Let's say we're looking at a new car and we decide that we want that car. If we really do want it, we begin to focus on it. More and more, we see it in our mind. We envision ourselves driving it. We can see the color, smell the new leather, and may even test-drive it. We begin to have feelings towards the car and talk about it. Unknowingly, and without really realizing it, we are beginning to synchronize our conscious and unconscious minds. We might draw the car, or cut out a picture of it and pin it in a place we will see it often. As time passes, and we focus more and more on the goal, each cell is aligning itself with the end result. And when all the factors throughout the body are aligned, something happens.

You may not realize the situation is connected, but it is. You may get a raise at work, or your old car may give up. Something will be the catalyst and you'll find yourself buying the car you have been thinking about for months. Now let's say you're going through the same process about something you do not want. Let's say you have a fear of being sick or having some specific disease. You begin to think about it and yes, you guessed it ... when you have thought about it enough and gone through the same steps, the conscious and subconscious minds come into alignment and the cells of the body will begin to comply. The cells are connected to the universe and have no judgment "as you will, so shall it be."

I don't know who first said it: "Be careful what you wish for ..." but truer words were never spoken. The art of manifesting what you want in your life has everything to do with focusing on the positive aspects of what you want. Maybe you are thinking right now, "How do we stop the negative thoughts? How do we not fear all the things that can happen?" Please know that the universe is always in balance. And so are we. There will be times when our thoughts are focused on the positive and times when we may slip into negative thought. This does not make you a bad person, or a negative person. Without the darkness, there would be no light. If we did not know sorrow, would we appreciate joy?

So when a negative thought comes, regardless of what it is, I recommend you embrace it. Smile upon it. Take it into your heart and find the origin of it. Just close your eyes and ask, "Where is this coming from?" You may be very surprised at what comes up for you. You may even see yourself as a small child. Your question may take you back to the origin of a blockage or a line of negative thoughts that have been with you for a very long time. Just close your eyes, take a couple of deep breaths, and wrap your heart around it. Embrace yourself and accept whatever it is that comes to you. Knowing that by accepting it and embracing it and thanking it, you may see it will just dissolve. The act of pushing the uncomfortable away or pretending it does not exist is what causes it to continue. When we own it, and honor it, the 'charge' on it may be released. Allowing it to be transformed into a feeling of gratefulness and joy. This is usually accompanied by tears, not of sadness, but of deep relief and thankfulness. This is the basis for the "ORT" process that will be the topic of Chapter 23.

I'd like to share this paragraph with you, even though the author is unknown.

"The ancients know the power of writing. They found that by putting in writing how you want your life to be, you reach past all fear and uncertainty into a higher realm of accomplishment. Through your definite written words, you dissolve all obstacles and barriers on the visible and invisible planes of life. Your written words go out into the ethers of the universe to work through people, circumstances, and events to open the way for your purpose and goals to become a reality." — *Unknown*

These words ring true, remember what we envision will manifest. So envision the life you have dreamed, let's create it now for ourselves, our family, our communities, our country and the entire planet. Below are 5 keys to opening the door to synchronizing your conscious and unconscious mind. This may seem so simple but it is true and does work: the more often you practice this the closer you become to your dream. *Close your eyes every day and see the dream as if it had already come true.)*

Five Keys to Manifesting:

1. Having the intention, seeing the outcome, and keeping it in the present tense.
2. Focusing on the goal; see it in your mind's eye.
3. Write it, draw it, and cut out pictures of it. The more media you have, the better it is.
4. Talk about it, share it, share the goal. Brainstorm about it.
5. Feel it in your heart. Feel the joy and the gratitude of it. Feel yourself being fulfilled in the present.

If you do these five steps at least once or twice a day, and keep the focus on the goal, you will be unconsciously aligning the conscious and unconscious mind, and as they become aligned, the cells of the body will act accordingly. And what you have dreamed about, and what you have desired, will manifest.

Chapter 14

Asking

So what do you want? What are you asking for? And the most important question, how are you asking? Most people I speak with want to be well, want to prosper and have a wonderful life filled with all the blessings of love and laughter and long life. "The good life," as they say. So what are you asking for? So many people I speak with are asking for strength ... I usually say rather alarmingly..."STOP! Do not ask for strength."

They look at me as if I am crazy but eventually ask, "Why?"

Well, here's why. First, I believe these universal laws were put here to remind us to stop expecting! Does spirit or God or the oneness or source (or whatever you humbly choose to refer to as your spiritual magnificence) owe us something?

We must put ourselves in the perspective of the universe. Now really think about this. What gives us strength? The trials, and the adversity in life, the challenges on emotional, physical, spiritual, mental levels. The misunderstandings, and the emotions that push us to the limit. These are what cause us to become strong. Remember that old saying: "What doesn't kill you makes you stronger." So when we ask for strength, we are really asking for more of the situations that make us strong, and give us strength. Some people say, "I've been praying for strength, and things just keep getting worse." I tell them, "Yes, of course they do! You're receiving *exactly* what you are asking for."

Chapter 15

The Hidden Blessing

It's important to understand that every moment is a blessing. Every moment is an opportunity because, even when the sky turns gray and there are storm clouds all around, there is still a blessing. It may not be always easy to see ... the loss of a loved one, the loss of a friend, relationship, countless events, countless things happen to each and every one of us as we grow through this human experience. As we find the blessings and begin to *act* in place of *react*, we begin to see the framework of our life begins to change. This does not happen in a day although it can happen in an instant.

For many years, I used to go to the prophet's conferences. It is a group of conferences held all over the country and around the world. It is a few days of up close and personal talks with some of the most brilliant minds on the planet. One year I was attending one of these conferences and Howard Martin, one of the founders of Heart Math, was speaking, and what he shared was very intriguing to me. Chapter 1 discussed how he showed scientifically that more signals go from the heart to the brain than from the brain to the

heart! The implications of this for me was very impactful.
Here's why.

Many think that the brain is running the show and for the
most part, that is so, or is it? If the heart is sending the messages to the brain that is letting the brain know how we are to
perceive any given situation, then we must ask, "Who is really
steering the boat?"

The answer in my opinion is the heart. This is also the
opinion of Heart Math. So you may be asking yourself, "What
does this have to do with finding the blessing?" It has everything to do with it. If our heart is feeling and perceiving and
sending the signals to the brain to act or react or not, then this
hearty little organ must somehow also be connected to the
unified field or non-local field. If the brain is taking instructions from the heart, then it is the heart that grows to the wisdom of any given situation.

Here is a true story I call "Soul Adjustment," for that is
what if felt like. I know now it was the point at which all the
knowledge I had learned to that point was turned into wisdom
and nothing would ever be the same. It was the most wonderful blessing any one could ever experience and I believe with
all my heart that this shift is waiting for each and every one of
us. And I know so many have already experienced this.

A few years ago, I helped create a Women's Empowerment
Group. My friend Sally and I spent much time planning and
organizing. We would take groups of women to a location in
the desert near Las Vegas and have meditations and do projects
that would lift each women's self-vision of herself. It was a
few years after my accident and I was still going through an

unwinding/rewinding process in my recovery. I agreed to do all of the cooking and the set-up. Sally, who liked to be in the spotlight, would do the meditations, etc. I was happy to stay in the background and be of service.

This was going very well and we talked with great excitement about franchising this and going from city to city and help to make a difference in as many lives as possible. On one of the weekends, someone asked me to do a Rune Reading for them. I did so and added some intuition and feeling I had about what I felt coming from the women's heart. She listened intently and began to sob and right there in front of me she broke through some suffering she was carrying and had been carrying for many years. I was taken back by the flood of e-motion but felt great gratitude to have helped this woman. It was one of my first clues that I myself had gone through an evolution of sorts. This was the last session of the season as the desert gets very hot in the summer and very cold in the winter. Our sessions were in spring. My partner and I set off in our own lives for a while. I was excited about the prospects of going other places and reaching more women, and could feel that I was finally beginning to reconnect to the world outside my own being. And perhaps in the process I would find my next level of service.

Some months later, as I was beginning to prepare for the coming season, I received a phone call from a mutual friend. She was excited on the phone, and I could hear her joy and enthusiasm coming loud and clear. She said, "I have some wonderful news. Sally has just chosen me to be her new partner in the Women's Empowerment Gatherings."

There was a moment of silence on the line. My mind began to race and I had flashes of all the pain and betrayal I had ever experienced in my life, and in that moment I knew somehow that this was an opportunity. I DID NOT REACT! I knew she had no idea what a blow she had just delivered. I took a breath and said genuinely, "I am so happy for you. I think this is a wonderful thing to be a part of!"

As I hung up the phone, I felt very strange, That instant of disbelief had taken the whole of the emotion and packaged it into a ball. I then proclaimed, "Okay, my heart, I know you are smarter than my brain, so you figure this one out."

It was the weirdest feeling, as if there was a floating ball of emotion around me, yet not in me. I was strangely calm and knew if I could find the blessing, the charge or the pain of the situation would just vanish. I had no idea what I was doing. I just felt as if I was following instructions. Were all the years of conferences, Kaballah, and hundreds of mystical and spiritual happenings finally coming to a head?

I had no idea if this would take an hour, a day a week or a year. I just walked around in this weird state. I felt as if there was some great work going on inside but it was none of my concern. (I know that sounds a bit crazy at best but it is true.) About three days later, I was walking into my hall way and it happened! In an instant, I felt as if the hand of source just reached into my heart and ripped out whatever mechanism it is in us that causes us to judge. It was so intense that I fell to my knees and began weeping, not in sadness but in joy. At first, I didn't know why I was sobbing but it was uncontrollable. I just wept and wept and then total bliss came over me and I knew the angels were very near. I felt such deep gratitude for Sally and the event that happened, I could hardly stand the beauty of it all. I knew in that moment I was not to stand in the background any more. I knew in that moment that each one of us is magnificent. My vision seemed to span the globe and I was just sitting on the floor, weeping, feeling the arms of the angels around me. It was as if I was let into some great secret.

It took a while for me to get up from the floor and as I did, I knew I had gone through an evolutionary leap of consciousness. I called it a 'soul adjustment' because that is what it felt like. I could hardly wait to call Sally and thank her. I was elated about this freedom and, in that moment, Inner Light Gatherings was born. I called Sally right away and was so happy I began to cry on the phone. I said, "Oh bless you for helping me, for being the catalyst that pushed my boundaries."

She thought I was being sarcastic and began begging for forgiveness. She said, "I am so sorry. I did not do this maliciously."

I kept saying, "No, no! Really, thank you. God bless you for helping me."

She did not understand why I was not devastated at what had happened. It took a while before she would even believe that I was so grateful for her actions. I felt so blessed and joyful and there was no trace of emotion or ill feeling. As the weeks went by, I noticed that as a situation would arise, I almost immediately would know the blessing, see the higher purpose and know that everything is always in divine order.

As we grow through our lives, sometimes we may be a catalyst for growth for others, just as others maybe a catalyst for growth for us. We dance this dance of cosmic ebb and flow with each

other in a continual motion and rhythm of life, as we know it
in this reality. Most of the time, we don't really know or understand what we may be for another being in the world of
actuality. As I look back at some event in my life where I may
have been harboring ill feelings for another, feeling somehow
unjustly dealt with, or playing the martyr part, I can now see
how each and every one of those beings was a catalyst in my
own evolution, a turning point for the unraveling of the mysteries of the universe. If we truly look at our lives, haven't
most of our creations come from some sort of disassembling
of what was the status quo? Some of us, maybe all of us, have
experienced total devastation of all that we knew and lived
for, only to find that we had been pushed beyond the limits of
our own existence. We were kicked out of the nest so to speak
and then we flew! We picked up the pieces and, if we truly
have healed and embraced the blessing of what was, we get to
truly move into what will be. It is time to move past the years
of healing and step into our true wellness – Our Intentional
Wellness.

Chapter 16

Who Forgives?

This is the age-old question that has been discussed through the millennia. It has been a common thread through every belief system, religion and spiritual practice.. "To forgive is divine" has been taught worldwide. We have been raised in a "You're right and I'm wrong," or, "I'm right and you are wrong," society.

I would like to offer you the opportunity to look at this in a new light. So take a deep breath, sit back and open your mind. I would like to share with you the thought that to forgive is actually a form of quiet arrogance. Now, before you jump out of your seat and react, let me explain.

Each and every one of us comes into this world on our own path, with our own life to create. With our own perspective on what is right for us. We move with the flow and energy of the cosmos. We encounter people through our life – all sizes, all shapes, beliefs, colors, creeds. As beings of light, it is really our job to accept and embrace those who come within our range or grasp. The very act of forgiving implies that someone is right and someone is wrong. If someone has hurt your feelings, is it really something they have done or your perspective of the situation and expectations about it. Is it really up to you to forgive?

I believe it is up to us as humans to accept one another exactly the way we are. And leave the rest to universal law and to spirit. It is time for each and every one of us to take responsibility for our own feelings and actions. If we are reacting to something, that is about our own perspective on any given situation.

It may be our job to be kind, to be understanding, to be a friend and to share views with other like-minded beings and beings who see things in a totally different way. Remember, everyone has a unique and different view of the world and everything in it. What is not our job is to change, alter or stand in judgment of any being or soul on this earthly plane.

Forgiveness is a quiet arrogance. Inside, if you search your heart, you will find that you feel a superior being-ness that allows you to feel you need to forgive anyone for anything. And since the events that occur in our life are merely opportunities from the universe, when we view these opportunities, we see that people, places and things are put into our life at exactly the right moment. So, I invite you to explore the possibilities. If you feel anger toward another, look inside yourself and see what event has been triggered. Who has caused you to become the judger? When we feel we have been wronged, more than likely it's a situation that has been set up by the universe for our benefit. We need only open our eyes and our hearts and then take an alternate route rather than reacting.

An example of this might be: One day Sally receives a call from a friend, Joseph. Joseph asks Sally to go to lunch with him. She says, "Yeah, that would be great." Joseph lets her know that he has to work until 2 p.m. and asks if a late lunch be okay.

Sally agrees to that. However, as noon rolls around, Sally begins to watch the clock. She begins to ask herself, "Why isn't he calling me? He said he would call. It's lunch time."

All these feelings come up. By 1 p.m., Sally begins to feel abandoned and is having feelings of inadequacy. By the time Joseph calls about 1:30, Sally is fit to be tied and says, "It's so late."

Joseph replies, "Well, I told you I may have to work until two."

Sally thinks about it and says, "Okay, I guess I could forgive you," as if Joseph has done something wrong.

The reality of the situation is that Joseph was a message from the universe. He merely did exactly what he said he would do. In his eyes, there had been no wrong-doing. This is an opportunity for Sally, who has some deep-seated issues about self-worth and abandonment. If she doesn't see the opportunity, it gets passed over and she will keep having the opportunity come up for her until she "gets it." Was there really any reason for her to forgive Joseph? Or was it her defense mechanism that caused her to cover up her feeling of inadequacy. Forgiveness is a quiet arrogance.

If we take it to heart that we are all beautiful divine beings and that things are exactly as we create them, our every action with everything, every moment and every event, and every interaction we encounter has been strategically placed for our benefit. Coming from a place of gentle repose, and looking deeper and beyond the surface situation, will take us to the place of truth and show us an opportunity to embrace and release that which inside of us causes us to react and causes us to falsely stand in a superior position where we feel we must forgive.

This is one thing I suggest you leave to spirit.

Chapter 17

Letting Spirit In

Do you speak about spirit as if it is separate and outside of you? Many people say, "It's difficult to get in touch with spirit," but the truth is, there is no need to try. Because we *are* spirits wearing skin, all you need do is close your eyes and come to the center of your feelings. Your natural state is that of continual connection, and all suffering comes from the sense of separation. When we feel separated from spirit, we feel separated from ourselves.

Like a giant grid throughout the universe, we are all connected. All of humanity, every plant, every mineral, every storm and every flame. We are all made from the elements and we carry the divine code within every cell of our body.

We are all connected and, in actuality, not separate or disconnected from spirit. For most people, this thought does not seem possible but I assure you it's true. When we use modalities or techniques such as meditation and visualization, we begin to see and feel that place of grace. It is in this place that we can clear ourselves and renew ourselves. We breathe in and visualize healing energy flowing into us, and breathe out and visualize all that no longer serves us leaving. Breathing in and visualizing our dreams, something miraculous happens. Every cell in the body hears that message and becomes awakened and open to the new feeling, and the new code is laid down throughout the cells. So the more we meditate and immerse ourselves in this spiritual body that we are, the more adept our cells become like exercising a muscle, and they begin to respond. I like to say: *"Meditation is a path to visualization and visualization is a path to wellness."*

When you ask the question: *Where does spirit reside?* the answer is that it resides within each one of us. When we spend time in nature and the elements, or sit on a rock or lie in a meadow and look up at the sky, or feel the warmth of the sun on our skin, we are opening our inner gateway to spirit and breathing in spirit. (I mention the elements because this is where we are closest to spirit.)

If you are willing, I invite you to try an experiment. Find a place that is comfortable for you. No matter where you are, you are always able to access your inner grace. If you can, take a walk in nature when you have some time to spend with your self. Go to the mountains or a place of nature by a river or by some beautiful pine trees. Find a place to lie down and get quiet. Begin to breathe in and release. You will find that in a very short time, you have been transported to a place of grace where your body seems to melt away and you become the nature that surrounds you. (It may take some time to be able to open to this kind of surrender, but every time you find the stillness, it becomes easier and easier to find your way back to this beautiful place of grace.)

Allow yourself to be touched by spirit. You will certainly be embraced by it, for it lives inside you. There is no separation.

You are spirit, and with every thought and every intention, your spirit will respond.

When you are grateful for all that you have and all that there is, your cells respond in a way that keeps this miraculous energy going strong. Intend to feel good. Intend to have purpose and wellness. Intend to live your dream. Breathe it in every day, see it, visualize it. Feel the joy in the moment and you will be amazed at how quickly the universe will comply. Let spirit in and know that it is and has always been there, deep within. Now it is your turn to embrace the wonder of who you truly are.

Chapter 18

Being Grateful

Somewhere between heaven and earth is a place so beautiful and so pure that when we arrive there, we often will have tears of joy. Have you ever had that feeling so deep in your heart – you know the feeling of total peace and joy, and you are so thankful for all that is – that tears stream down your face and all you can say is, "Thank you, thank you, thank you."

Every feeling we have has a coinciding frequency. Love and the feeling we have when we're in love create a very high frequency. So does gratefulness. Being grateful is one of the highest frequencies we know of at this time. It's right up there with prayer. Being grateful is a key component to Intentional Wellness. So how do we get grateful?

So many people seem to see all the things they do *not* have, rather than seeing all that they *do* have. In every moment, we have an opportunity to be grateful. Grateful for the breath that we're taking, grateful for the vision that allows us to see this beautiful world. Grateful for the heart that allows us to feel wherever you are at and whatever condition you may be in.

Beginning to find that place of gratefulness is the beginning of the place that you will find wellness. Being grateful in the moment — always in present tense — is a key element to shifting our consciousness, to aligning our conscious and subconscious minds, and to begin the process of realigning the cells of the body. I'll share with you a little morning and night ritual I have found very effective.

Every morning when I first open my eyes, the very first words out of my mouth are, *"Thank you for this glorious day, thank you for the perfect health, and the perfect wellness I experience. Thank you for the love and respect of my friends and family and community. Thank you for the abundance and the prosperity in my life today. Thank you for allowing me to walk in spirit. Thank you for allowing spirit to move through me. And thank you for going before me and making my way that I may walk in my highest good today."*

These words are spoken *every morning* before I rise, and *every night* before I close my eyes to go to sleep. You may choose to find your own words, but I highly recommend this as a daily ritual of being grateful.

"Gratitude opens up the gateway of your heart and lets your ever-present love radiate out and shine. Your heart just loves. There is nothing but love all else is illusion."

— Dr. John Demartini

Chapter 19

Power of Intention

"Intention is the beginning of the outcome"

— Sheila Z

Through our intention, all things may be created. Intention is the link between the realm of possibilities and the reality of creation. Through intention, we all have the ability to bring forth information from a unified field to what we know as reality and actuality. If we go back and take apart the action of intention, it would be like unraveling the fabric of time and space. Like taking apart a magic act that causes life itself to manifest and flourish.

Does intention come from universal information? Or does intention begin within our very own heart and soul? That's the question many people seek to answer. It is the intention that can move mountains. It is your intention that can take you beyond any limitation. When you see your dream within yourself and you feel it, you begin a cellular reaction that puts the wheels of the universe in motion. It is your intention to follow your dream. It is the intention to bring your dream into the realm of reality that becomes the driving force. It is something we cannot see or touch, yet the reality is, the energy of intention is what drives all life on this planet. Without the first intention, there is no movement. When a child looks at a chair, sizes up the chair, sees itself grabbing onto the chair and pulling itself up, it is the intention that drove the action and the child is standing. It is the same mechanism that allows us to get up from a fall, to think and believe and hope of a better future.

It may be indeed the power of our intention that will put into motion the reorganization and implementation of a new way of seeing our own beings as the instrument of health and wellness, of peace and prosperity and as stewards of this great and precious earth. As more and more people become awake and aware that their every thought, their every intention, has an effect on the "all," we are beginning to realize we can guide our intention and so guide our thoughts. Like a finely woven fabric, we interweave into our own future. We see it, we feel it, and it touches all of our senses. The power of intention is within each and every one of us. It has always been there, awaiting our glance.

Unconsciously, we are creating intention in every moment. That is why it is so important that we are in touch with our intention, our true intention. That we look at everything in life with profound gratitude. Coming from that place, our intention can be the driving force for the realization of all of our dreams.

Intention is there before the thought. Therefore, it is the intention that we are learning to work with. My statement: "Our intention is the beginning of the outcome" is true indeed. And the intention, our intention, is one of the most profound forces in the universe. It is time for us to see and feel how we fit into the universal plan. Time to see that All That Is is by the intention and action of those who have gone before us. It is now our time to step up and be the universal beings we are designed to be. To use our hearts and our intentions and our free will to heal the past of this earthly plane, to see and think and feel the bright and glorious future awaiting each and everyone of us. To love, honor and respect this beautiful planet we call home. As we nurture the earth and all her inhabitants, so our own health and wellness will emerge like a new spring flower. There is not a moment to waste. Now is the time to intend the brightest future for us all.

The ABCs of an Intention Driven Life:
* Activate the healer within
* Become your fulfilled potential
* Create your intention

Chapter 20

The Healer Within

The concept of the healer within is not new, only forgotten. "Natural forces within us are the true healers of disease," spoken and written by Hippocrates (460 – 357 BC). Let's think about that for a moment. This means that 460 years before the birth of Christ people knew they were the driving force in their own healing and wellness. So what happened?

Through the ages, there have been healers, those who heard the call, in tribes and clans. Before this time there were medicine men and women, elders and wise ones. There were shamans and healers and teachers of the old ways.

As we entered a time of patriarchal society there came a new word: "physician." Before this were medicine men and women, elders and wise ones. The age of science ushered in a man's world, and the women in the healing profession became nurses and assistants to physicians. Like the good father, the doctor would tell you what to do and what to take to help you to recover from whatever was ailing you.

Somewhere along the line, we as a society began to distance ourselves from our own health and well-being. We just live our lives and if we get sick, we just go to the doctors and do what they say. In this country, the age of taking responsibility for our own well-being ended about the same time the pilgrims' boats landed on these beautiful shores.

I am in no way dismissing or putting down the medical field, and the men and women who dedicate their lives to helping the rest of us to maintain health and so live a fulfilled life. I am suggesting that, somewhere in this process, doctors became like gods, the absolute end all in healthcare. Just take a pill and feel better became the status quo.

In today's hustle-bustle world, most people rely on others to tell them what to do and how to take care of themselves. And many have become very dependent on what others say is the best thing for them.

Well, the buck must stop here. Taking control, doing your homework, gaining knowledge and wisdom on the workings of your own being are finally emerging as more and more important, as people are beginning to realize that they themselves must take responsibility for their own wellness. (The 45 million Americans without health insurance know this only too well.)

We are explorers by nature, always seeking more and more truth, a better way and a better life. Your quality of life has a direct relation to your perspective and your willingness to seek that which pushes you into the place of a universal being. Taking the reins and knowing you are the creator of your future goes a long way to being ready, willing and able to seek the optimal you. Your best life is right now, right here and in every moment hereafter. You are the healer; you are the prophet; you are the one you have been waiting for. Now is the time to claim it, be it and live your dream.

In This Moment: Timeless Healing

Quantum Physics says we are holographic beings, and that each cell remembers. In this energetic adventure, we explore how to read universal and timeless energy, to heal and be healed in the body's present moment. Journey to the beginning and look into the eyes of the child, a remembering of angel glow. Through love and acceptance, you may be guided to release cellular imprints that no longer allow access to your true and optimal self. Recapture the grace and fullness of authentic selfhood.

New Knowledge and new tools are being introduced every day. The future of medicine may very well be sound and vibration. As we learn more about our molecular structure and see that we are made of sound and vibration, I feel with certainty that in the future when we have an organ or a part of us out of alignment, in distress or dis-ease, we may place the correct frequency on the outside of the body and the organ will come back into balance.

Breaking the sound code is the next step in our medical journey. Already there are tools such as Acutonics[1] that may heal with sound and vibration by utilizing universal aesthetic energy and placing it on the key meridians point of the body. These tones are familiar and reside within each of us. We are gaining the wisdom to look through a clearer lens and envision all that is and all that will be. This is an exciting time to be part of the evolution we are all experiencing – the awakening and re-awakening to the "Healer Within."

---

[1]   In this modality, tuning forks with carefully selected frequencies that have been calibrated to the planets are placed on the acupuncture points on the body and clear the meridians and energy pathways.

Chapter 21

Doorway to Connection: Putting It All Together

All through this writing there have been many different thought footprints and a diverse array of paths and perspectives. We have explored the physics of our form and the science behind some of the newer methods of self-exploration and the exploration of wellness as it pertains to our own life. So now we have many pieces of the puzzle, how do we connect them to bring about the activation of the higher frequencies and so bring into view an expanded perception of our life and the gateway to a future of perfect health and Intentional wellness?

The good news is it has already been pulled together, just as your entire body is made up of thousands of different pathways that all interact and share connections and work together in a symbiotic relation. Take breathing for example. Just breathe in ... now let's take a look at what just happened. As you breathe in, the cilia (tiny hairs) in the nose begin to filter out particles, the cells are alerted of the incoming oxygen and every cell responds as the lungs fill. The bloodstream absorbs oxygen and the brain is revitalized with the incoming life-giving element of air. And then, as miraculous as it came in, we exhale and expel the carbon dioxide our bodies cannot use or assimilate. However, the plant life on this planet lives and thrives on this carbon dioxide and takes it in, turns it back into oxygen and expels it … and we breathe it in. How's that for a symbiotic relationship – and a very good reason to be sure that the plant kingdom on this planet is happy and thriving, for we are directly connected to their well-being. Yes, the miles of veins and arteries and 100 trillion cells are all reborn with every breath we take in. It seems like an impossible mission but it is all put together without us having to consciously think about it. It's the same when we breathe out or exhale. All the used molecules are drawn from the cells, organs, muscles and tissue, and expelled into the atmosphere. Then the cycle begins again.

So it is with information. When you read the words or look at a picture, the information goes through every cell and is stored within the body. Every word is assimilated and the body responds. You may feel happy or sad or excited or mad. We all have a symbiotic relation with every moment of every moment.

The information you have been reading is already assimilated and your body, mind and spirit are already able to use the knowledge and wisdom from everything you take in. It is cumulative in that it all adds up! That is how we change and grow. That is a key component to our conscious evolution. It is happening right now! Congratulations! It will be used in your highest good.

The doorway to connection lies within you. Just inside your vessel, just behind your eyes. It is always there, the great doorway to your authentic self. We must close our eyes to see it. We must breathe in the energy, the prana, the chi of life to activate it. We go within to the awakened dream, to the center and from that place, we can be immersed in the light of pure gratitude and joy. We can embrace and release that which keeps us from our fulfilled and optimal self. The doorway to connection is within each and every one of us. It was placed within, hiding in plain sight. Safe and always present. This is the place we can dance with our soul; this is the place we can view and activate Intentional Wellness.

Chapter 22

Meditation and Visualization

"Meditation is the pathway to visualization ,Visualization is the pathway to Wellness"

— Sheila Z

If you are one of the many thousands of people who meditate on a regular basis, I salute you. For most people, the word "meditation" brings up visions of far off temples and monks quietly sitting by a tree in a beautiful green meadow. It implies something far away and Eastern in origin. Meditation is the most ancient form of prayer and is not necessarily a religious practice although many religions have adopted this form of quiet connection to source. It is more of a spiritual and self-exploring practice. If we look back in history, we will see that most religions had some sort of meditation in its daily practice.

There are many forms of meditation, and everyone can benefit from the practice of meditation. In our very hurried and rushed modern day living, it is difficult to even think about making time to quiet the mind and relax the body. Everyone is capable of meditation and anyone can do it. More and more, it has become clear that meditation has a profound impact in a positive way in the area of wellness for the person who make the time to meditate.

The statistics are astounding – upwards of 30 to 40% fewer heart attacks for people who meditate. And if you happen to be in the hospital, the statistics show if you meditate, you will have about a 30% faster recovery. So something is going on and that something is connection to self and source. For some, it may be the art of mind over matter but it is far more than that. It is actually the art of the no mind and all heart, exploring the vastness of your yet-to-be-discovered self.

It is a beautiful way to enhance your creative self, find clearer focus and promote a healthier and happier life. Meditation has been an expanding practice whose time I believe has finally come.

Meditation is described in the dictionary as: *(verb)* "to think deeply or focus one's mind for a period of time, in silence or with the aid of chanting, for religious or spiritual in purpose or as a method of relaxation."

Visualization is described as: "the process of creating internal mental images (internal visualization and imagination) and the engaging of one's imagination within the body-mind to effect changes in consciousness."

I find this a bit contrary to how I describe meditation. For the purpose of healing and raising one's vibratory rate, the one thing we do not want is to stay in the mind. Meditation is about getting a distance from the mind and exploring the inner feelings and realms of the heart and soul. It is from this vantage point that we may glimpse the divine, and it is from this vantage point that we move from meditation to visualization. Meditation is the process and practice of quieting the conscious mind, traveling to uncharted territories, and allowing our spirits to soar with the angels and feel the light of spirit.

There are many types of meditation. For our intent and purpose I would like to talk about Visionary Meditation:

In visionary meditation, we explore and create places usually with a purpose. We visit what I call "the valley of the Spirit." Each individual will have a variation of the same journey, which is perfectly fine as our lifelong influences and belief systems will have some effect on the journey. As we grow and blossom, and evolve as human beings, our experiences in the meditative state will change as well.

This valley of spirit is a trail head, a place from which we venture out. In a visionary meditation, we may be seeking an answer to a question or seeking wisdom. We can ask questions of our guides, our angels and our optimal self. Yes, from this place we can connect directly with source.

Some of my own experience with visionary meditation has been extraordinary. I have been able to travel to the past and venture to the future. I have visited with departed spirits and ascended to a place of the divine self. Carrying a grateful and joyous seed in my heart has been the key that has opened many of these doorways.

The Foundation and Practice of Meditation

As with any healing technique or practice, a commitment of will is certainly one of the foundations of meditation. This is a commitment to one's self and one's optimal self to keep an open heart and an open mind to the inner wisdom that may come forth. The practice of meditation requires the will and desire to discover that which lies awaiting within. As a healing practice for both the self and others, this is a powerful practice of which every human is capable. Once you have tried this calming and rejuvenating practice, you may feel beckoned to continue. Your body may be asking you to listen to that which lies within. Your heart may be waiting to reveal the secrets of the universe and the pathway to better health and wellness. Your spirit may be calling for you to awaken that which has been asleep. Or you simply might be curious about how meditation can enrich the quality of your life.

Meditation is quieting the conscious mind. "Why do we want to quiet the mind?" you might ask.

There are several reasons to quiet the mind. My personal favorite is that when we quiet the conscious mind, we allow our true inner self to travel to places that are inaccessible to the fully conscious and waking mind. When we quiet the mind, we open a doorway to the subconscious mind. We can travel to inner worlds as, when we are in meditation, a portal opens before us and we can step onto a path of discovery and we can access our cellular memory. In this place, we can promote healing and wellness, not only for the self but also for all beings and for our planet. I know from experience that meditation and visualization are doorways to other dimensions and one can pierce the veil through this practice.

We can access and remember the wisdom of the ages that I believe lies awaiting in each of us. In this place of quiet repose we may find the doorway to our soul.

Chapter 23

Opportunity Retrieval Technique (ORT)

What is ORT?

ORT is a process we can experience for the purpose of achieving cellular release. It is really a form of cellular re-patterning. I use the term "retrieval" because opportunity is always there. Every moment the universe is bringing to us opportunities of every kind, size, shape and color. We may not always see it as opportunities but that is exactly what they are. Opportunities and blessings in the fabric of the energy weave us and connect us to each other and to All That Is.

Many paths may lead to a given goal. It is becoming very clear that the frequency of the human species is rising and wonderful paths are opening up everywhere we turn. It is as if the universe has opened up and sent forth the message that it is time to be well and understand what unique and beautiful beings we truly are, awakening to the expanded self that lies within.

We come into this world a unique and precious soul. This does not change. Our angel glow can last up to a year or so but usually fades by about 7 months. As we begin to fit in to our new human life form, we see, hear and soak in all that surrounds us. Our needs at that age are great and we rely on our source figures, our family. There are many who will say, "Well, I did not really have a family." When I talk about source figures, I am including anyone and everyone who had a hand in your care and your early years.

Many techniques will say, "Leave behind all that does not serve you." Or, "Push away or make powerless that part that is causing you stress or disease." I differ from belief, as I believe we all came into this world with all of the information we need to grow into the magnificent beings we are. All parts of our being are intricate and vital to the whole. Yes, all 100 trillion cells have a unique and yet congruent job to do. From every cell, there are signals and impulses that create the who, the what and the why of our being. I believe when we embrace that part that is out of alignment or, in a state of dis-ease we have an opportunity awaiting to open, one that may bring this part, this cell, this area back into alignment and balance, and back to wellness.

To truly love and honor all of your being, embracing and feeling on a cellular level that you are in alignment, and when the cells truly believe and feel this love and acceptance, this allowing, this embrace, we may experience a transformation, a healing, a re-awakening.

I would like to say this is easy and all we have to do is love ourselves through and through, and indeed this would be true. We have all heard of miraculous healings and some of us have actually witnessed this. There is much more to this than meets the eye, however, because what we are saying on the conscious level, or thinking we believe on the conscious level, has little to do with the actuality that our subconscious mind is really running the show. So what is your subconscious mind saying and believing? That is the real question. All the events and all the systems that live in the subconscious will determine how and what you feel, and how you heal.

So why don't we always see these opportunities?

Our bodies see, hear, smell, taste and feel everything we come in contact with. Everything is recorded and stored in our cells. There are times in our life from birth to crossing that we are unable to address some data we have taken in. Our body stores this data until a later time when we are hopefully better equipped to handle the information. This stored information has a profound effect on our perception and our behavior. It is the information we use to make our choices in life. It is what has molded us, and our experiences play a major role in how we grow and what we will experience in the future. It then becomes very clear that to update the files and release the old information is key in maintaining health and balance in our life. That is why I call these files Pockets of Opportunity. As I mentioned in Chapter 7, these pockets remain until we go back and release the file. In essence, we retrieve the opportunity that was offered to us regardless of the time that has passed in between.

Here is an example: A dear friend of mine stopped by one day and was telling me how angry she was at a business associate. "She just pushes my buttons and I am very angry and upset."

I explained that this was a good sign and a wonderful opportunity to clear an old trauma off every cell in her body. She looked at me as if I were a bit daft but agreed to try anything that might help. I asked her to close her eyes, take a few deep breaths and connect to her heart, to the truth of the feeling. I asked her to ask, "Where is all this anger coming from? Please show me the seed of this."

She closed her eyes and in a few moments opened them and said, "Oh my God. I saw myself as a 12-year-old girl and I was violated by a friend. It wasn't too traumatic, so I decided to just go on as if it hadn't even happened."

I asked her to place herself in a safe place with her offender sitting across the room from her (he was behind a rope and so could not harm her). Then I asked her to tell her offender how it made her feel and how she would have liked it to be. As she spoke, tears came to her eyes as she felt the confusion and anger she had been holding on to for so long. Then I asked her to allow him to speak. Her offender began to weep and beg her forgiveness. He said, "I was abused as a child by my father, and my life was one of anger and pain. I have thought of that day for years with horror and regret."

His tale was so compelling that my friend began to weep with compassion for this poor soul and in that moment the trauma poured out of her, the feeling of true compassion released the anger and shame from every cell.

For me the question is, wherever this person may be, did he receive the healing as well? Since the sequence of this method takes us for a few moments out of the timeline and into the non-local, my feeling is yes, the healing when a full release is complete encompasses all parties involved.

This means that whatever situation or person is triggering you is really presenting the opportunity to go back and release the file. When we are ready, the opportunity will show itself. We just have to be aware that this indeed is an opportunity. My friend got it immediately and even though we didn't do a full release on it, just having the information began to unravel the patterning. She called me the next day to say how different she felt and how she was able to handle the situation differently. Her perspective was shifted ever so slightly, and she began to see the blessing of it and be thankful for the situation that had been the catalyst for the release. It is the feeling we are after, the feeling we go back to. And the release of the file raises our frequency and so our perspective.

The technique is very simple, however I highly advise the first couple of times you experience the "ORT" process, you do so with a skilled facilitator or at an Intentional Wellness Conference. I believe it is with the non-blaming or what is called the "benevolent witness" that we are more able to release and re-pattern. It is through a relational event that this pocket of opportunity was stored, so it is most effectively released in the same way. After experiencing this a few times, you may find yourself going through the steps on your own, you will have the knowledge and will be able to go through the steps on your own if you so choose. Remember, the universe never gives you more than you can handle. Just know when a situation arises – whether it's anger, resentment, jealousy or feelings of betrayal – it is these emotions that are triggered by pockets of opportunity that are ready, willing and able to be released.

The steps to the "ORT" process are:

1   Stay in the feeling.

2   Take a few deep breaths.

3   Close your eyes and go to your heart.

4   Ask, "Where is this coming from," or, "Show me the origin of this feeling."

5   A picture, a name or a face will come up. Sometimes emotion comes up. Whatever it is, know you are safe. See yourself telling the person how their action caused you to feel. I like to begin with, "You hurt me when …."

6   Tell them the way you would have liked it to be, and how you would have liked the situation to have been handled.

7   Then allow them to speak. See them understanding what you are saying. And know most of the time, they have been suffering from this incident as well. See their loss and confusion. When you find yourself having compassion, you are ready to seek the blessing.

8   Find the blessing. Think about how this helped you in your life either to gain more understanding or compassion. Or has this made you a survivor, stronger and more able to handle your situations? When you truly see and feel the blessing, something happens. Your heart opens and you begin to weep with gratitude for the event or situation. As the tears flow, the file is dissolved. The pocket disappears and every cell in the body releases its piece of the memory and you are freed and uplifted to a higher vibration, a higher frequency.

From this point on, you will be able to see this much clearer in all facets of your life. As you use this process, you may also begin to feel lighter, more alive and well. You will have a sense of empowerment and know you have a tool to help create the wellness in your life you have always intended. You are creating Intentional Wellness.

Chapter 24

You Are The Light

It's in the Light:

"Each of us is a living being. As such, the most obvious fundamental medium of our connection to the universe is light. Even the simplest fungus or protozoa has receptors that respond to the presence of light. The most feared thing about imprisonment, or even death, is the loss of contact with the light. Light is the ultimate source of life. Without the light coming from the sun, there would be no life here on earth. Light is not only the only medium of contact with the world, in a very real sense, it is the basis for our existence. If the difference between us and dead matter is organization, it is sunlight that provides the energy and impetus for the self-organization of matter into life, on every scale, from the individual cell to the life of the whole planet and from my morning awakening to the whole history of evolution."

— *Lee Smolin Ph.D. Prof. of Physics — Penn. State Univ.*

Yes, you are the light. Each and every soul illuminates the time and space it occupies. Your physical form is the temple you chose to experience this realm this time around.

117

This is your time here and now. Every moment of every day, you have a choice to shine as it was intended to be. You are the creator of your world and you choose how you view it. You also have the choice to view yourself as only a pawn in the game of life, allowing what seems to be reality to push and move you at will.

Are you holding on to that which will cloud your true view of your own light? Are you beginning to see you have the opportunity to go through your "files," those pockets that make the path way back to your true angelic glow?

Every blessing you see and feel, every blessing you realize, puts you at the gates of the next opportunity. Find your passion. Do what you love and love what you do. Allow your light to shine.

Just by being you every moment of every moment, you help others to be who they truly are. Knowingly or unknowingly, how you walk in this world will serve to inspire others and help hope to live in the hearts of all you encounter.

Know in your heart and soul how beautiful you truly are. Close your eyes often and feel the light of spirit shining on you and through you. "Intend to feel good." Every day, practice the "Being Grateful" ritual. Practice random acts of kindness. This is how it was intended to be. This beautiful golden woven fabric that weaves its way through time and space. You are a part of it all. We are all a part of it all. This writing has touched on many pieces of the "Earth experience puzzle" and, like a puzzle, the more pieces we have in place, the clearer the picture becomes.

It is time to Seek the Soul and Heal the Body. Step into the illuminated being you were always intended to be and are. With your intention and your light, you can open to the miracles that are always surrounding you. The time is here, the time is now. The pages have been written; there is no time to waste. You are a vital and important part of this entire planet going to the next level in health and wellness. Feel the light from within, dance and play in the wisdom of who you are. Laugh and love with all your heart. Kindle your flame, your passion for this life each and every day.

You are the light; You are the light; You are the light,
We can all see you shining.

Chapter 25

Stories & Testimonials

This section of the book has six sections of testimonials and stories:

1. From listeners of *Sounds of the Soul*
2. From meditation with *Sounds of the Soul*
3. From hands-on healing sessions
4. From the Intentional Wellness all-Day Conference™
5. From the "ORT" process:
6. From the author:

From the moment *Sounds of the Soul* came through me, it was evident that the tones and frequencies within this channeled piece of music were having a profound effect on many who would hear it either in passing by or in a session with me. The music was a big piece of the puzzle that facilitated my own healing and enhanced my connection not only to the angelic realm and the realm of the divine but also facilitated boundryless travel and exploration of my spirit and soul.

Please know that these testimonials are just a small sampling of the overwhelming transformations and grateful response from those who have been touched by *Sounds of the Soul*. They were sent by individuals who felt compelled to share their story or feelings.

Section I: Testimonials and stories from listeners of Sounds of The Soul.

Sheila Z -

I want you to know how special and profound the music you channeled, *Sounds of the Soul* has been to me. This music resonates at a levels that opens my heart and soul to realms that seem so expanded - my mind loses its place to "think." The words "spirit eternal within the body" bring me back to my center of being, oneness, vastness, blissed and eternal.

I have never been moved by such awe inspiring music. I want you to know it is one of the few things in my life that is constant, "spirit eternal" and it is *the one true thing* that helps keep my life in balance. Every night as I go to sleep, I use headsets so I hear and feel the experience of a this multidimensional reality taking me way beyond what we might consider the norm of reality, into a world of love and peace, from the inside out!

Sounds of the Soul is angelic and one of the most peace-filled, soul expanding experiences I have ever had ... and I have had many, in many realms.

I am honored to share *Sounds of the Soul* with everyone I know ... and I have experienced *Sounds of the Soul* does not necessarily resonate with everyone even though it could. The seeming fact is, not everyone opens their heart and relieves their mind chatter in the same way. Some cannot stop their mind, some do not hear the multidimensional levels, some are not able to hear dimensions of the music, and some cannot even hear the words, and the words are so profound...

The magic is, *Sounds of the Soul* resonates on different frequencies depending on the resonating frequency of the listener ... I am blessed to soar to blessed-filled, creative states with

the music; others might want to consider losing their mind
chatter a little and open to the power of their universe within.
There is nothing more awesome then *being at one with eternal!*

Blessings to this music – it has wings for the soul.

All the best,

Namaste.

(This is from a family who used Sounds of the Soul *to help a
loved one cross peacefully)*

Remarkable,

I can't let another day go by without telling you about the
remarkable passing of my brother-in-law, Bill, in S.D.

When we went to see him, he was very weak and so close
to death I didn't know if he would make it through the day.
However, I put on your CD *Sounds of the Soul,* and Bill fell into
a very deep restful sleep, and he seemed to be quite peaceful.
It appeared he was sleeping quite well, so we slipped out without bothering him when we left. The next day when we arrived, I was happy to hear he still had the music playing. Matter
of fact, it had not stopped all night! We talked to him and this
day he seemed stronger and more awake. We spent about 2
hours with him, then he fell asleep and we left. The next day
when we returned, we visited for about an hour, He was awake
and able to speak a little. We brought him a chocolate milk
shake and he consumed it with pleasure. We said our good-
byes and on May 2, Bill went to be with the Lord.

The next day, Bill's wife called us to ask if she could keep
the *Sounds of the Soul* CD. She explained that for the entire
time since we left, Bill had it playing, When she came in some
days, it was turned up so loud she could hear it down the hall
as she entered the building. Bill kept his window opened and

she could hear it as she walked up to the building. Needless to say, she saw that it gave Bill great relaxation and comfort, and she wanted to connect with those days of releasing and acceptance for him and the transition into eternity she felt these sounds helped him to achieve. One more thing, as he entered into the fast breathing stage as he neared death, someone had turned down the music so you could hardly hear it. When Bill's wife came in, she turned it up, and in just a few minutes, his breathing slowed down and it appeared his heart quit racing. Also, he became very calm and peaceful.

So thank you, Sheila, for being a willing servant to bring into our lives the blessing of your song, sounds that give help and hope. Thank you.

Sheila,

I want you to know what an incredible difference your music *Sounds of the Soul* has been for me and how it has truly affected my life. From the first time I listened with headsets, the multidimensional sounds of your angelic voice awoken up the deepest part of 'Self,' the IAM.

Sounds of the Soul takes me deep into self and off to universal wonderland. My sleep is so sound, and I also listen in the morning for meditation ... it sets my day off in peace.

I can only touch on what it has done for my deep sense of well-being.

Sheila Z's *Sounds of the Soul* CD has inspired me on so many levels. The first time I meditated to it in Sheila's class, my angels and guides appeared. I knew I had to buy the CD. I listen to it every day now when I am meditating. I have always received some type of vision or message when I do. It is angelic sound-

ing, and it elevates and expands my energy. Even my house-
plants have responded positively since I began playing it!

Your music CD is amazing! Every single time I listen to it,
I cry. Not tears of sadness; more like tears from feeling I'm in
the presence of my own spirit/greatness and I am completely
humbled by this loving reunion /contact with my authentic
self or Spirit.

The first time I heard your CD was at the Summer Sol-
stice, June 2005. After meditating with *Sounds of the Soul* gen-
tly playing in the background, my whole body was tingling. I
felt a clearing of my energy and a surge of creativity unlike
anything I have ever experienced before. I was compelled to
start painting and drawing, not something I usually feel compelled to do. That wonderful feeling lasted two weeks! I knew
I had to have this CD in my collection!

I suffer with migraine headaches and try to stay away from
prescription drugs as much as I can. The very first time I heard
Sounds of the Soul 1, the notes soothed me immediately and
started to take the edge off my headache. Now at the very
first signs of a headache, whether I feel sick to my stomach or
have visual signs, I put on Sheila's CD and close my eyes. The
beautiful music and her angelic voice have helped me avoid
the use of drugs many times and I have been able to resume
my normal activities.

Section 2: Testimonials and stories from meditations guided by Sheila Z with Sounds of The Soul.

Meditation Session:

Sheila, in writing to you about the meditations, I am finding myself examining the experience from a different stand point. I had no idea how thirsty I had been for the comfort, caring and all the other feelings I was enveloped in. Finding all this out in meditation is a beautiful experience. Each meditation is different. I am looking forward to the next one.

After my session with you, I felt so much lighter, peaceful and energized. I felt so lost and directionless before our session. It was as if I wanted to jump out of my skin and run away but I didn't know where to or what from.

After our session, I felt comfort I knew I was going to be just fine no matter what path I took in my life. I felt I was shown or given a doorway and when I was ready, all I had to do was turn the handle and walk through itl which would lead me to the pathway of my highest good.

Remote Meditation session:

I was in the hospital and Sheila sat in healing meditation for me that evening and sent me remote healing from her home the night before my procedure. The morning of the operation, I woke up after sleeping in the hospital very soundly. (This is unheard of for me.) My husband commented on how relaxed I was. And I really was.

I know it was the energy sent by Sheila the night before. She has a wonderful gift of healing. I highly recommend her. Her meditations are as healing as her hands.

My extraordinary experience during a meditation with *Sounds of the Soul* was at our last G.I.F.T.S. Party. I had been feeling a little tight from asthma during the party. As we were finding a comfortable place to meditate, my chest was so tight and I was wheezing up a storm. I didn't want to get up and disturb everyone so I just started to listen to the wonderful tones and echoes on the CD. After a couple of breaths my chest simply lifted and opened! My lungs felt clearer than they do after I take my inhaler! Wow!

I would like to tell you about my experiences with Sheila's guided meditations. I moved to Las Vegas in early November and asked the Universe to send me people of "like mind." Well I received this blessing with much gratitude, as it led me to Sheila.

I went last night, after waking up with a headache (I am not a headache person!) that had continued the whole day. I also had dislocated my little finger on Sunday and it was swollen and painful and I had a splint on it when I walked in. Sheila guided us through the first meditation knowing I had a headache (thank you Sheila) as the headache dissolved.

After the break and the second meditation, my finger was vibrating, along with the rest of my body. There was no longer any pain or swelling and so I took the splint off. It is still feeling much better today and still no splint! In fact, I am still vibrating today and it feels wonderful. What a blessing to find Sheila. I am curious to know where our journey will lead us. I know I am in the right place. Thank you for sharing your gifts with us. You are wonderful and I think you should tape all of your meditations and sell them! Really I do.

Dear Sheila,

I feel compelled to share with you my experience of the meditation on February 18, 2005. First, I always enjoy your guided meditations. Your focus, awareness and joy of meditating are tangible. Your presence radiates peace, calmness and serenity. I thank you for entering my life.

The meditation of Friday the 18th was especially moving for me. As you guided us into the valley, I felt not only a peace within but also a part of the group. I felt that all our energies were linked together. I was also able to visualize us, individually and as a group.

You do know I have had a block with visualizing in meditation. What a wonderful treat, to be able to visualize. During the part of the meditation that the Golden Energy was showering us with the healing energy, I felt the rain of energy splashing against my body, feeling as if I were being showered with sparkling water. My whole body was tingling. I remember an almost giggly sensation, just like being a child. I even turned up my face to get more.

You guided us to remember someone who loved us, and I thought of Sandy, my husband. I then felt my heart and soul being *touched* with kindness, compassion, warmth and love. It was as if a part of my pain/grief/defenses/whatever had melted. That *touch* was so gentle it brought tears, not my normal tears of weeping. These tears just kept coming and coming in a steady stream. I did not even think to try to stop them; I gave into the process, as completely as I could. I did not even know just how protected and comfortable my pain was. It has been a part of my being for such a long time. Until, it started to melt.

As you were bringing us back, the colors started. The green was a rich, deep, dark, silky green that swirled and almost danced. It was almost like seeing a long-lost friend. There was a sense of recognition and joy. My heart smiles at the memory.

Little did I know, there was yet another gift. The colors blended and kept changing from green to gold. As the colors were rippling upwards, there were faces there. The faces had dark eyebrows and dark hair. They had the most compassionate eyes, and the gentlest of smiles. The faces were oval. As one traveled upward, another one appeared, and then another. I don't know how many there were, more than one, less than twenty. It seemed as if they were happy I was aware of them. I was delighted to see them. Then we came back.

Oh Sheila, since Friday (it is now Tuesday) I have been seeing the world through expanded senses. Senses that have become more aware of the people and the world around. There are even periods of joy, a joy that has eluded me for so long. A joy that is welcomed in every cell of my being. I feel that my prayers are stronger and more focused.

I have never even known what my deep-seated dreams or desires were. Now, I stand a chance of finding out. An unexpected door is opening. Isn't life wonderful?

Gratefully yours,

Section 3: Testimonials and stories from people whom have experienced a hands-on healing session with Sheila Z

I had an old shoulder injury that bothered me much of the time, and had gotten used to it. I did Reiki on it, stretching, etc. Sheila offered to see if she could help me, and she removed the pain almost immediately. I felt it leaving my body. The pain was gone and has not returned. It has been over 3 months now!

Dear Sheila,

I want to take the time to thank you so very much for what you and your open heart did for me during the session you so freely gave of yourself and spirit.

As you are aware, I had just been involved in a serious car accident that knocked me unconscious, knocked the wind out of me, bruising my ribcage and internal organs, as well as having the air bag totally burn the skin entirely off of my left hand from the nitrous oxide that it lets out upon exploding. I would not have received the burn but because I was knocked out cold, my left hand remained on the steering wheel so I did not feel it being burned. It was not until I awakened in the ambulance strapped to a board with an IV in me that I began to feel pain.

I was off work for two days and when I returned, you happened to call my office regarding the Beauty, Health and Fitness Expo we were putting on at the Cashman Center. Before I even realized it, I was sharing my horrible experience with you and you offered me an "alternative healing session." I was a little weary but concerned because my burn was not healing at all and all the doctors had offered were cream, coverings, and pain pills. Since my burn showed no signs of even trying to scab or heal, I made an appointment with you. This was the most wonderful appointment that a doctor could never offer.

I arrived at your home a little hesitant and instantly you made me feel safe and comfortable. When you took your rock around me to cut all strings, cord, and attachments not for my higher good, I thought this is interesting. However, instantly, I felt a freedom and security I had only one other time known a long time ago. Then you pulled out negative energy and I felt it coming out of the soles of my feet and somehow you knew exactly where I needed it. Then you began filling me with healing energy and when you came to my left arm, it felt like my wrist opened up and my left hand became warm and tingling. I had not even noticed that I had felt disconnected from my injured hand until it opened and the tingling and warmth penetrated into it.

I suddenly knew I was loved, and tears of joy came down my face. I was connected again to my source, my universe, and my heart was open. That warm feeling of being one and connected and loved swept over me. Unless someone experiences this themselves, it is very hard to describe.

The next morning, I took the bandage off my hand to change it and, to my surprise; it was covered with a thin layer of skin! No scabbing, just a thin layer of skin and everyday it thickened. It never scabbed and it is now totally healed. When I returned to the doctor for my check-up, he was amazed. He could not believe his eyes. No scabbing, infection or anything he was expecting. It was healed.

Words can never express my gratitude to you for the work you do. Thank you from the deepest part of my being for being who you are and using the gifts you have developed to help me and all the others you will help.

Sheila,

Having a healing session with you was an incredible journey into bliss. Your intuitive touch was like having someone who could really see and feel my energy and knew how to move and release the denser energies. I went from being stressed to very relaxed and feeling at peace. It feels like you are in an angel realm when you are doing your healing work, truly like you are in tune and care about the whole person on many levels.

Thank you for being you.

Dear Sheila,

Thank you so much for healing my foot – really my toe but it affected my entire foot. Three weeks ago, I was bitten several times when I accidentally stepped in an area swarming with ants. Strangely, everything was on one toe and there was one main bite and several smaller ones. My toe became immobile and stiff. It was three times the size of the other toes which had also swollen. Soon after that an angry red area appeared and was working my way up the ankle.

Clearly it was infected and all the over-the-counter stuff I bought at regular and homeopathic pharmacies was not working. I called you to see if there was anything you could do and you suggested that you do an intuitive touch healing on it.

I could feel the banishment of the infection as you worked over me for about ten minutes – the power was literally palpable. When I left your office, I could wriggle my toe and felt somewhat better. I felt good in general with the expectation that my toe would heal. Previously I was in a lot of pain and concerned because no other methods worked.

That evening my toe began a spontaneous draining that lasted for three days. More and more stuff emerged and the site became a gnarly bump with an eventual scab. This was definitely not pretty but it was not red. My foot returned to normal size within two days of your touch and the redness abated almost like the tide washing out to sea. Every few hours, it slowly retreated.

Truly, those who saw it could not believe the astounding difference. Thank you again, it was a miracle.

Sincerely in awe,

I had been feeling pain the area around my solar plexus for quite a while. It had been a constant pain, a feeling of "fullness" and really annoying. It was at the point sometimes that I really couldn't even eat, I was so uncomfortable. Then one day, I actually pressed into the area and was amazed how much it hurt to press on it. It was more painful on the left side than on the right. I was thinking I'd finally have to go to a doctor to see what was going on, but not really happy about that because, then they send you to a "specialist," etc. I also thought the pain was a combination of both the physical and emotional.

I was at Sheila Z's house to do some work together and I told her what was going on. She very kindly said, "Well let's see what we can do about this." I had never had any kind of sound healing done on me before and I didn't really think getting some "vibrations" would do all that much, but figured, I really had nothing to lose and Sheila was so willing to help. I lay down on her table and she just did what she does for a few minutes. I thanked her and left, not really thinking much had happened and/or helped.

The next day, however, I noticed it was a bit better. By 72 hours later, the pain and discomfort were COMPLETELY gone. I can now press really hard into the area that I could barely touch and there is absolutely no pain. I am very familiar with all types of healing methods, but this is the first time I had experienced anything like this. For me, it was a miracle. I am extremely grateful for Sheila's generosity and intuitive touch.

After a session with Sheila, the vertigo I had been experiencing for the past four years was dramatically decreased. I had no signs of it for days and it has improved.

Section 4: Testimonials and stories from participants of the Intentional Wellness™ All-day Workshop

Sheila Z's "Intentional Wellness" workshop is on the cutting edge of healing and of health and fitness, in that she offers an enlightened holistic approach supported by the latest in scientific research. It seems that even in the world of fitness, in which I have worked for more than 18 years, there is a need to understand that the road to getting into shape begins with intention., This experience with which Sheila Z provides you that resonates in your body on a cellular level, and as a result, you are changed. Sheila Z assists you to move from a place where health and fitness are just out of reach, to feeling and experiencing the state of wellness in the present moment. In making that shift, you are already on your way to achieving your goals, whatever they are. It is obvious to me that Sheila Z is one of the enlightened ones of our time who is shedding light on the truth about who we are, the power we all have to transform ourselves, and our true connection to our bodies. Thank you again for sharing your enlightened approach.

We had a wonderful time at the Intentional Wellness Conference Saturday and feel so enlightened by the energies that surrounded us that day. You were magnificent and we so appreciated the time you spent personally with us on a few issues. Thank you so much for a truly joyous day! We hope to see you in the future, and until then, may the white light shine upon you and yours.

Sheila,

THANK YOU! What an incredible experience! I love you! Thank you Universe! So the day itself was incredible because I met a few people who I instantly felt a connection to. The rest of the day, I felt soooo centered, balanced, connected to spirit and "plugged in," as I like to say. I went to my friend's house and she commented that I looked different, "prettier." During the ORT, when you asked us to think of a trauma we would like to heal, I immediately thought of abandonment, of how the woman who gave birth to me left me for my grandparents to raise; but I thought that was too deep a subject to get into, but I could NOT think of another trauma! And when another lady in the group brought up abandonment, I took it as a sign and decided to try and work through it. When I told Pat how I felt and listened for her perspective, all I heard was, "I wasn't meant to be a mother" and I got stuck in that moment and couldn't move forward." I wanted to hear your thoughts on this, but then we broke up into groups, which at first I was a little disappointed about, because I thought I was there to hear from the "master," not the other students. In retrospect, the other group members brought up things and said things that clicked in my mind and were helpful and wouldn't have been brought up with just one-on-one interaction with you, so it was all just perfect!

Also, I went to my friends' house and I was sharing with them what we did in the conference, and I just started telling stories from my past and healing traumas I hadn't even realized were traumas! This morning when I woke up, the first thing I thought was. "Thank you, Universe, for my perfect health, for this great day." It was just a really great experience and I will most certainly be at the next conference! Thank you, Sheila! Thank you, Universe!

Sheila,

What a BEAUTIFUL day! If I do nothing else just for me this year, I will still glow from this experience for a very long time. I awoke the next morning to an almost electric energy pulling me so high up and so refreshed! I know you understand without my explanation. Thank you again so very much for sharing the gifts the Universe has placed in your care. You are a wonderful vehicle for all that positivity to travel to all corners of the world.

Sending You Light and Love,

Section 5: Testimonials and stories from those who have experienced an "ORT" session

Sheila!

What a great session it was! You helped me silence all the outside influences and hard-wired expectations of myself and realize that it's finally OK just "to be"!

Spirit and my Father look at things through an eternal perspective. I need not rush the second half of my life! I can simply be grateful for what I've learnel deposit all the lessons in my "archives of learning" and start anew! YAAAAAAYYY!

It is indeed your connection with spirit and my willingness to succumb which together helped me achieve this epiphany. I did not expect to be taken back to that sweetest of all places in my youth where I pocketed my innocence, never EVER to be the same. And yet I AM! I am back where I started yet much stronger and wiser! What a cherished gift!

Thank you! Thank you! Thank you!

Section 6: Testimonial and story from the author

I know I told the story about myself in the beginning of this writing and I do not want to be redundant, but I must say, I am so grateful for the gift I have been loaned from divine spirit and for being taken in and held in the arms of the angels. I am walking, talking, breathing, singing, dancing, loving and joyful proof that Intentional Wellness can bring you from any state of being into a state of harmonic balance.

I was given the clues to create this for the lifting of the frequencies of all humans. I myself spent months just listening to *Sounds of the Soul* day and night. When I would be in a place almost too unbearable to go on, I just put on my head phones and did a healing on myself. I am so healed and well that I make a joke of it, with, "I do not look good on paper but I am perfectly well." But it is not a joke. It is the truth.

With being diagnosed with so many injuries, including the traumatic brain injury, I know in my heart I am a miracle just as I now know we are *all* the miracle. I wrote once, "In the moment of no more moments, the angels came," and I meant it. They would take me by the arms and pull me from the depths of my delusion and we would soar. They saved me many times over. The angels are a continual presence in my life. I am walking in the prayer. I am keeping my promise to spirit do dedicate my life to the wellness and the healing of humanity and to our precious mother earth. I thank you for being a part of the awakening, the birthing of the future.

In gratitude and the brightest of Blessings.

Epilogue

Dear Ones,

We are living in the time of the great awakening. Perhaps a time of re-awakening. For years, we have felt the push of the energies of conscious evolution as our planet and our civilization are reaching out for the next step in the universal plan. We are birthing into a new way of life on this planet.

I have come to understand that this evolution is indeed spiritual in nature. We are spiritual beings; each of us in our own spiritual awakening, individually emerging into a higher vibration, a new view of life on this planet a knowing and a feeling of certainty that All That Is is really from the light, and in every moment, we really are being given opportunities to grow into our divine self.

How we choose to go forward from here will have a direct impact on the future of this planet. Yes, we have entered a time of consequence and the clock is ticking and pushing us to evolve with the intense energies that are building. The year 2012 is a blink away and we all now have the opportunity to flourish and embrace the transformation at hand. Make the Leap. Activate your future self. Live and be your dream and highest vision, now. Take the journey to Intentional Wellness and live in Joy and fulfillment from this moment on.

My deepest love and gratitude for each and every moment of this glorious life.

Sheila Z Stirling

Glossary

What is "Spiritual Evolution?"

Spiritual - If we look at the literal meaning, Webster's describes *spirit* as: "the breadth of life, the soul." And *spiritual* as: "as or pertinent to the spirit, like the soul, to sacred things."

Spiritual is that which we may not be able to see but it is the core of who we are. When we hear a piece of music that is so beautiful it brings tears to our eyes, that is spirit in action. When we comfort a friend with sincere caring and compassion, that is spirit. When all seems to have forsaken us and we stand alone in the darkness and hold on to that small spark of everlasting light that is the core of who we are, that is spirit. To believe and know with certainty that this is only the beginning and that every moment, we are given the opportunity to step into our fulfillment, that is spirit. When tears roll down our cheeks with gratitude, and the beauty that is this life, that is spirit. It is all around us, it is within us; it is the essence of who and what we are. It is the reflection of the divine that lives within each living life force; every creature and every living plant has a spiritual connection, a higher purpose flowing through this realm in perfect symmetry, perfect timing, the seasons, the tides, the wind and the rain, the warmth of the sun and the sweet earth beneath our feet. In that precious moment when the miracle of life emerges into this world, that is spirit and in that moment, we know we are all the reflection of the divine.

Evolution: Webster's describes *evolution* as: "to exhibit or produce by evolution; to become open, disclosed, or developed; to unfold." It is the last word of Webster that I would begin with, for evolution is the unfolding. We must be open to unfold. As the earth herself grows and changes, so each of us has been evolving since the dawn of time. Regardless of how we came to be in this paradise, whether it was from the sea to the land, or from a distant place, the moment we became a part of this garden, we began to grow in every way. As we developed, we used our free will to ever expand life on this planet. We are expanding now every nano-second. We reach for the next step in our evolution. I believe we are at an extraordinary time in our evolution, a time of great expansion, new dimensions, new paradigms and a new way of being. Those of us who are answering the call push to the next level, soar with the angels and be the change and live the change for the betterment of the planet and all who dwell here. That is evolution. To know with certainty that only with honor and mutual respect for every living creature and all of nature, will we be able to go forth as intended. To allow the old way to fall and step into what will be. To step with kindness and compassion, with a heart expanded to encompass all of humanity and all the elements. Now you're talking evolution.

Bioenergetics: Wikipedia, defines *Bioenergetics* as: "a field of biochemistry that concerns energy flow through living systems." This is an active area of biological research that includes the study of thousands of different cellular processes, such as cellular respiration and the many other metabolic processes that can lead to production and utilization of energy in forms such as ATP molecules. All biological processes, including the chemical reactions of bioenergetics, obey the "laws" of thermodynamics.

I recently read this description of Bioenergetics: "Pertaining to human health from a perspective of interactions with externally applied electro-magnetic stimuli, either as a matter of intentional modalities or environmentally imposed factors."

Interpretation by Sheila z Stirling:

Our bodies are made up of hundreds of systems. One very basic system is that we are electrical in nature. If a heart stops, most of the time it can be restarted with an electrical charge. In many countries today, they are using electricity to detect "diseases" as anything in the human body that is out of harmony will have an altered electrical pattern. Bioenergetics is an alternative healing modality whose time has come in my opinion. When we listen to music, it affects us on a cellular level. It is altering the electrical signature and can be seen and so proven on modern medical equipment. When we have intention as well as stimulation such as sound, we are indeed using bioenergetics to bring about optimal health and wellness.

Neuroenergetics: This pertains to the mind and the neuro pathways that guide our every move – miles and miles of nerves and neurons that take in and give out information to the body on a cellular level. When we meditate or do a cellular re-patterning, it is actually the neuro cells we are seeking to transform, to release trauma from the neuro pathways and so bring the flow of energy "life" back into harmony.

Boundryless: This pertains to the full experience of non-confined space and time.

Opportunity Retrieval Technique (O.R.T.): This is a proprietary technique created by Sheila Z Stirling. O.R.T. is an emotional intelligence and re-patterning method where, while in a waking meditative state, you travel back to the seed, blockage, or a Pocket of Opportunity. This technique allows you to get back to the feeling that caused the cellular disruption and re-pattern it for the purpose of releasing the trauma from all the cells in the body and thus removing any further or future damage that may occur in any and every area of your life.

Allopathic Medicine: As defined in Wikipedia: "Some medical dictionaries define the term *Allopathy* or *Allopathic medicine* as the treatment of disease using conventional evidence-based medical therapies, as opposed to the use of alternative medical or non-conventional therapies

"The term allopathic, an adjective, is used in medicine to distinguish one form of medical practice, medical tradition, or medical profession from another. The term was coined by the founder of homeopathic medicine, and was used through the 19th Century as a derogatory term for the practitioners of orthodox medicine. The meaning and controversy surrounding the term can be traced to its original usage during a heated 19th-century debate between practitioners of homeopathy, and those they derisively referred to as 'allopaths.'

"Today, the term 'allopathic medicine' has been revived and its use as a synonym for mainstream medicine has become common. In recent years, many M.D.s accept this designation, i.e. an 'allopathic physician.' In the United States, 'allopathic' is used by the American Medical Association, the National Residency Matching Program, and the Association of American

Medical Colleges. These organizations use the term to distinguish the schools and residency training programs which they govern from the osteopathic medical schools and programs, accredited by the American Osteopathic Association."

Homeopathic Medicine: Was created in the late 18th century by a German physician named Samuel Hahneman. The remedies can be made from substances that, if undiluted, may cause symptoms similar to the ailment they were given to treat. At this point, there is a great controversy going on about the effectiveness, meaning and practice of homeopathy. The legal status of homeopathy varies from country to country, (as stated in Wikipedia) but homeopathic remedies are generally not tested and regulated under the same laws as conventional drugs. Usage is also variable and ranges from only two percent of people in Britain and the United States using homeopathy in any one year, to India, where homeopathy now forms part of traditional medicine and is used by approximately 15 percent of the population. Flower remedies are a part of homeopathy, and are produced by placing flowers in water and exposing them to sunlight. The most famous of these are the Bach flower remedies, which were developed by the homeopath Edward Bach. The relationship between these remedies and homeopathy is controversial. On the one hand, the proponents of these remedies share homeopathy's vitalist world-view and the remedies are claimed to act through the same hypothetical vital force. However, although many of the same plants are used as in homeopathy, flower remedies are used undiluted. There is no convincing scientific or clinical evidence for flower remedies being effective. (Many people claim to have had healing experiences and so an open mind is essential when investigating and using alternative healing modalities.)

Naturopathic Medicine: as defined in Wikipedia: "Naturopathic medicine (also known as naturopathy) is a school of medical philosophy and practice that seeks to improve health and treat disease chiefly by assisting the body's innate capacity to recover from illness and injury. Naturopathic practice may include a broad array of different modalities, including manual therapy, hydrotherapy, herbalism, acupuncture, counseling, environmental medicine, aromatherapy, nutritional counseling, homeopathy, and so on. Practitioners tend to emphasize a holistic approach to patient care. Naturopathy has its origins in a variety of world medicine practices, including the Ayurveda of India and Nature Cure of Europe. It is today practiced in many countries around the world in one form or another, where it is subject to different standards of regulation and levels of acceptance.

"Naturopathic practitioners prefer not to use invasive surgery, or most synthetic drugs, preferring 'natural' remedies, for instance relatively unprocessed or whole medications, such as herbs and foods. Practitioners from accredited schools are trained to use diagnostic tests such as imaging and blood tests before deciding upon the full course of treatment. If the patient does not respond to these treatments, they are often referred to physicians who utilize standard medical care to treat the underlying disease or condition.

Emonopathic Medicine: This term was created by Sheila Z Stirling and refers to the practice of healing the self. Naturopathic, homeopathic, and allopathic all use outside procedures, tonics, pharmaceuticals or plants all which reside beyond the body, beyond the self. Emonopathic goes within, and with specialized techniques, may be effective in healing the body, mind and spirit from a cellular level. The blending of ancient ways and modern methods has proven to be very effective.

Osteopathic Medicine: This is defined as hands-on medicine that looks at the whole body and corrects problems caused by musculoskeletal imbalance – an inter-relationship that is the emphasis of the osteopath.

According to Wikipedia, it is defined as: "a branch of medicine based on the premise that the primary role of the physician is to facilitate the body's inherent ability to heal itself. Though practiced mainly in the United States, osteopathic medicine shares a common historical origin with a type of complementary medicine practiced worldwide, known as osteopathy. Physicians who graduate from osteopathic medical schools are sometimes known as osteopathic physicians and hold a doctorate in osteopathic medicine (D.O.)."

Other Creations from
Sheila Z Stirling

Reading the Language of the Cosmos

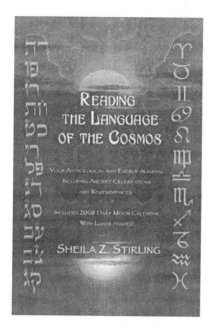

Motivational Astrology - This book is a channeled work that explains the energy and influence that surrounds our world on a moment to moment basis. A detailed description of the energies of each sign of the zodiac and examples of how that may affect your life, plus an interesting interpretation of Kabbalahistic Astrology. At the back of the book is a daily moon chart for each month of the year, including phases of the moon and a chapter on how to deal with and be better prepared as the lunar energy comes into play in our every day life. A brilliant and captivating book that makes your life more joyous and fulfilling.

Lynne Palmer, world renowned astrologer, gives this book a big thumbs up, stating, "It is well-written and a must for anyone who is seeking a happy and productive life. The author believes that we are in an evolutionary leap and this information has been out in the cosmos since time began. Now is the time to seek this information for the highest good and betterment of all."

Sounds of the Soul CD

Sounds of the Soul was channeled from the celestial realm. Cutting edge scientific studies are now being done with neuro-feedback EEGs and the initial findings are astounding. This CD when listened to through headphones seems to balance Alpha, Beta, Theta, and Delta brain waves. The implications of this are boundless and, as we know, meditation has the ability to decrease blood pressure and stress levels. We also know that *Sounds of the Soul* may potentially normalize brain function and, in doing so, heal the body on a cellular and soul level. Open your heart and breathe in the music.

Sounds of the Soul was channeled through Sheila Z in collaboration with Gary Stadler of Heartmagic Studios, and is an interpretation of the God code of creation. The sounds and tones are very relaxing and channel directly to the soul. Many have experienced a reconnection with spirit and accelerated healing.

There are 2 tracks on this CD. One is 18:50 min and the other is 27:24 minutes.

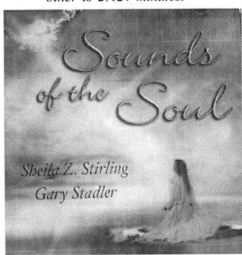

To order, please go to: *www.OpenWisdomInstitute.com.* Click on Books & CDs, or Store, and listen to a free clip of the CD. $15 plus $5 shipping within the United States.

Healing Meditation
with the Sounds of the Soul CD

This is a journey meditation that encourages your connection to the healer within. Building the healing energy of the cosmos an being in the heightened vibrations of the angelic realms from Sounds of the Soul.

This meditation is about 27 minutes.

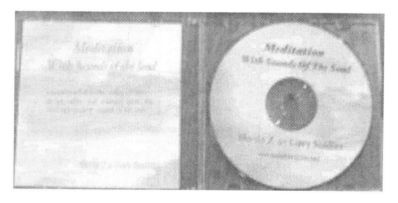

To order or comment, please go to the web site:

www.OpenWisdomInstitute.com.

$15 plus $5 shipping within the United States.

LaVergne, TN USA
07 April 2010
178408LV00002B/8/A